LIZ EARLE'S
QUICK GUIDES

Aromatherapy

D1350143

BⓈXTREE

ADVICE TO THE READER

Before using essential oils or following advice on aromatherapy contained in this book it is recommended that you consult a doctor if you suffer from any health problems or special conditions or if you are in any doubt

First published in Great Britain in 1994 by Boxtree Limited, Broadwall House, 21 Broadwall, London SE1 9PL

The right of Liz Earle to be identified as Author of this Work has been asserted by her in accordance with the Copyright, Designs and Patents Act 1988

10 9 8 7 6 5 4 3 2 1

ISBN: 1 85283 542 7

Text design by Blackjacks
Cover design by Hammond Hammond

Printed and Bound in Great Britain by Cox & Wyman Ltd., Reading, Berkshire

A CIP catalogue entry for this book is available from the British Library

Contents

ACKNOWLEDGEMENTS

I am grateful to Sarah Mobsby for helping to produce this book. Also to professional aromatherapists Jan Kusmerick, Geraldine Howard and Pat Suthers. I am also indebted to the talented team at Boxtree and Claire Bowles Publicity for their unfailing enthusiasm and support.

Introduction

Welcome to the wonderful world of aromatherapy. I have been using essential oils and aromatherapy techniques for many years – not only for myself, but also for the health and well-being of my whole family. With the help of this *Quick Guide*, you will find that the art of aromatherapy is quick and simple to learn. This book gives you all you need to put the principles of aromatherapy into practice. Before long, you may even wonder how you ever managed without these aromatic essences and the many benefits they bring to both mind and body. I hope you enjoy exploring this fascinating natural therapy for a long time to come.

Liz Earle

1

The Ages of Aroma

The art of aromatherapy is nothing new. In fact, the use of essential oils to restore the physique and soothe the psyche is almost as old as civilisation itself. Aromatherapy has withstood the test of time and some of the modern-day remedies and recipes are the same as those thousands of years old.

The Ancient Egyptians were among the first to use fragrant oils for bathing and massage. This was advocated nearly 6,000 years ago by a physician called Imhotep who was later deified as a god of healing and medicine. Fragrant essential oils were just as important to them in life after death and were given as offerings or for the afterlife. Many aromatic essences and essential oil containers were found in the tombs of King Menes (about 3000 BC) and the famous boy king Tutankhamun.

Essential oils were also an important part of life in ancient Greece. Sweet smells were attributed to divine origin. In the myths gods descended on scented clouds wearing robes imbued with aromatic essences and the eternal afterlife was reputed to be perfumed by scented rivers. The Greeks also made sophisticated use of aromatic substances, both for cosmetics and medicines. One ancient manuscript reads, 'The best recipe for health is to apply sweet scents to the brain.'

Around 400 BC, Hippocrates, who has been called 'the father of medicine', recommended the use of fragrant baths and scented massages on a regular basis for good health. He also used aromatic fumigations in the streets of Athens to help stem the spread of plague. In the second century BC, a physician called Asclepiades believed in the soothing, healing and curative properties of bathing, massage, perfume, music and wine – the ideal life-style perhaps? Yet another Greek, Theophrastus, made the astute observation, now scientifically proven, that oils applied externally are absorbed through the skin into the bloodstream and affect the body internally.

The Romans inherited this knowledge of aromatherapy, and so it spread with the Roman Empire. We all know about their love of bathing (hence the city of Bath and other spa towns), and their extravagant use of fragrant oils. The Emperor Nero's love of aroma was so great that he installed in his palace a system of pipes to blow out perfume-laden air – rather putting the modern-day air freshener to shame. Nero even covered himself with an entire year's supply of perfume at the funeral of his second wife Poppaea. Perfume can also be credited with changing the course of history as Mark Antony was said to have been intoxicated by the scent of rose and patchouli oils on Cleopatra's skin!

With the decline of the Roman Empire, the use of fragrant essential oils in the Western world was reduced and the knowledge was lost. In India and China, however, the traditions of the natural healing arts have remained unbroken. In India the use of plants reflect the religious and philosophical view of man as a constantly changing process of nature. Ancient texts have been found containing formulae and even invocations to the plants themselves; 'Come, you wise plants, heal this patient for me', is one such example.

While Europe abandoned bathing and fine perfumes during the Middle Ages, an important breakthrough occurred in Constantinople at around the turn of the tenth century. The discovery of distillation meant easier extraction of essential oils and far greater purity than was possible with the previous methods. This discovery is widely attributed to Avicenna, although in reality it was developed over a period of time. Drawings of essential oil stills in Arab manuscripts reveal that the original method of distillation is exactly the same as that used today, although with slightly less sophisticated apparatus.

Essential oils were brought to Britain with the returning Crusaders and became popular not only as perfumes, but also to ward off the plague. Queen Elizabeth I was a great believer in perfumes (not surprising, given that baths were a rarity) and she copied Catherine de Medici's habit of wearing scented gloves, although she did not emulate Catherine's 'gifts' to her enemies of poisoned gloves. Soon the British court was smelling sweetly of rose, lavender and jasmine – thanks to the aromatic essential oils.

Such an influx of knowledge led to the publication of 'Herbals' which were collections of recipes and methods enabling the women of households to make their own infused oils, aromatic waters and decoctions. The herbs themselves were used to scent bed linen, clothing and even the entire house. Herbal mixtures were strewn on floors to deter rodents, and made up into pomanders or bouquets to ward off infection.

In the seventeenth century, herbalism reached a peak, with famous names such Culpeper and Gerard researching and writing their works. Essential oils now formed a small but regular part of the herbalists' remedies, and the names of these influential men have survived into the twentieth century, with the Culpeper herb shops in our high streets and Gerard's range of herbal remedies still available today.

Alongside the development of herbalism, the seventeenth century also saw the early beginnings of experimental chemistry and with it the birth of scepticism for natural remedies. Over time these were virtually dismissed as superstition or 'old wives' tales' and were replaced by synthetically produced drugs. The deadlock was broken when the Frenchman Gattefosse burned his hand in a laboratory explosion and plunged it into the closest liquid, which just happened to be pure lavender oil. His hand healed remarkably quickly with no infection or scarring.

This led him into researching the essential oils and their many beneficial properties. In fact it was Gattefosse who invented the term 'aromathérapie' in the early 1930s. He wrote a book by this name, which remains in print today and is still referred to widely by practising aromatherapists.

During the Second World War a French army surgeon, Dr Jean Valnet, also experimented with aromatherapy. He used essential oils as antiseptics on wounds with very good results. Valnet also observed that those soldiers living and sleeping in pine forests suffered fewer colds and common respiratory disorders. The only factor to which this could be attributed was the scent from the trees – a case of natural aromatherapy! Valnet's great interest led him to carry on using essential oils after the war and he included them in his work on psychiatric patients. This was a great success in spite of the initial scepticism of the hospital staff. Dr Valnet was an extremely important contributor to the scientific validity of aromatherapy and his research papers are still valued today.

Another great innovator was Marguerite Maury. She probably had more to do with aromatherapy as we know it today than any other person. This is because she was one of the first, with very few exceptions, in almost a thousand years to combine the use of essential oils (diluted with vegetable oils) with the techniques of massage. Madame Maury studied the penetrative powers of essential oils and proved that they had both quick absorption through the skin and highly effective results. She also introduced a more holistic approach and the notion of individual prescription of essential oils. She was a woman of amazing energy and dedication who practised, taught and wrote until her death at the age of seventy-three – her last manuscript on aromatherapy was found by her bedside.

Tiny acorns grow into great oaks. Likewise aromatherapy has spread from small beginnings. Now a common treatment in France, the use of essential oils is included in the curriculum of some medical schools. In other countries, even industry is beginning to utilise the benefits of aromatherapy. Some Japanese companies now use their air conditioning systems as giant diffusers, and are dispersing energising oils into the atmosphere to invigorate the workers. Here in Britain, aromatherapy has become far more widely accepted and is being used by many nurses in conjunction with conventional medicine. The NHS area health authorities have even started to appoint Consultant Clinical Aromatherapists. Perhaps one day in the future we will see a fully qualified aromatherapist on every hospital ward.

The popularity of this therapy, which is still in its infancy, can be seen by the rapid rate of growth, both in the numbers of people visiting qualified practitioners and in the huge increase in sales of essential oils. And every day still more people are discovering the bountiful benefits and delights of this ancient art. Not long ago, very few had even heard the term 'aromatherapy'. Now the proven pleasures of aromatherapy mean that the art of using essential oils for health and beauty is here to stay.

— 2 —
What is Aromatherapy?

Aromatherapy is a natural therapy. It uses the fragrant and powerful essential oils to treat a wide range of physical and mental problems. Treatment of the whole human being – body, mind and mood – is very important as the physical body and the mind's psyche are closely interlinked. A change in one greatly affects the other. In addition to the specific medical uses of aromatherapy it is very useful to promote general health and well-being. Aromatherapy is a truly delightful and enjoyable therapy for people of all ages.

The Dual Action

The essential oils used in aromatherapy work in two different ways. Firstly, through the sense of smell, and secondly, via absorption into the skin. The sense of touch is also important and the medium of massage is an integral part of aromatherapy.

AROMA
All smells, pleasant or not, are a continuous part of our environment. Each of us has an emotional and instinctive reaction to them. We can say immediately whether we like a smell or not, yet trying to describe one is immensely difficult. The words used to describe fragrances often do so by reference to something else and then only outline the type of smell rather than the specific, for example floral, spicy, green or exotic. Although smell is probably our most underdeveloped sense (in relation to its

capacity) we use it more than we realise consciously. It actually accounts for around 80 percent of what we would term 'taste'. The sense of taste itself is an incredibly blunt sensor and the subtleties of flavouring from our food are more often picked up by the olfactory system in our nose.

Smells can also have an effect without us realising it. Although many products on sale obviously are perfumed (we often choose our shampoo, or indeed a washing powder, by whether or not we like the smell), some products are perfumed to such a small degree that we may not be aware of it. Experiments have shown that consumers prefer the scented article to an identical unscented one. Many shops and restaurants put the aroma from their kitchens and bakeries to work in the selling department – pumping it around to just outside the entrance, we are enticed in by our noses! Supermarkets frequently waft the aroma of freshly baked bread across the bread counter. Nature also puts a high value on the sense of smell: it is the first sense to exist in primitive organisms and the last to leave a dying person.

Our sense of smell has a profound and immediate effect on the way we feel. This is probably because smells access the brain directly, particularly that part which is the emotional hub of the human being. This direct link begins with nerve endings having direct contact with the outside world. Approximately 800 million nerve endings are found in the thin sheet of membrane covering the olfactory organs, located at the top of the nose. Their only function is to detect smells. It is interesting to note that these nerve endings are the only set we have which are self-replenishing – all others gradually deteriorate over time. The 'scent messages' are then sent straight to the brain through the olfactory system. In the brain these are received by the limbic system, a part of the brain responsible for controlling our moods and emotions. The limbic system has a huge memory capacity, being able to build up a library of millions of different smells. Nothing evokes a memory more effectively than a smell – a whiff of suntan oil can transport you instantly to a tropical beach, or the scent of freshly cut grass may bring back childhood memories in a flash.

ABSORPTION

Essential oils have a very small molecular structure which enables them to slip through the skin. They are quickly absorbed into the bloodstream – it can take as little as twenty minutes from application for the essential oils to enter the bloodstream. The oil molecules then travel the entire body via an intricate network of blood vessels. This means that they are able to work on the whole body and all its systems. Finally, they are excreted from the body through the natural methods of urine, sweat and breath exhalation. This process takes six hours or less in a normal, healthy person and up to around fourteen hours in an overweight or unhealthy body. This extraordinary ability of the human body to absorb substances through the skin can be seen in examples of conventional medicine where a drug or hormone patch is stuck to the skin to pass the substance into the body.

Absorbtion of essential oils through the skin is a very powerful way of treating the body. Partly because the essential oils themselves are so powerful and have many varied properties. All are antiseptic, some are antibiotic, others antifungal, antiviral, or anti-inflammatory. Some essential oils can stimulate the circulatory system or the lymphatic system and they can also activate and strengthen the body's own natural immune system. Essential oils begin their work immediately, first on a patch of skin, then working more deeply in the area and organs directly beneath the application, and finally throughout the whole body. This means that specific areas can be targeted while still treating the body as a whole; all without having to go through the digestive system. In fact, essential oils are medicines which work more effectively when absorbed through the skin than when taken orally (never take essential oils by mouth except under the guidance of a qualified practitioner).

TOUCH

Massage is the most important and commonly used medium of aromatherapy. It utilises the dual action of smell and absorption of the essential oils to its utmost and has a great 'feel good' factor. Not only this but it exploits fully the healing power of touch. This is no myth, but a natural instinct in all of us. We instinctively rub a bump, bruise, or area of stiffness on ourselves to ease the ache or pain. If someone else is in pain, be it physical or mental, our natural reaction is to give them a hug or simply establish some form of contact, even if it is just by touching their arm. Children are far less inhibited than adults and will even hug themselves when distressed. On the scientific side, it has been shown that touch causes the brain to release chemicals called endorphins which are the natural pain-killers of the body. Our sense of touch is not simply a healer, but also necessary for general good health. It has been proven in studies that children who are regularly touched are actually healthier. Consider the importance of contact between mother and baby; if denied this (or similar contact with another person) babies can actually become ill. This need for physical contact remains with all of us throughout our lives. Massage is therefore an immensely useful form of touching. Massage is also especially useful for those who are uncomfortable with physical contact and avoid touching others, as it provides a more formal framework for that contact. This is especially true when visiting a qualified aromatherapist where there may be a degree of anonymity. We should not forget that touch is one of the greatest forms of communication that exist. Between the extremes of making love to that of punching someone's lights out, there exists a whole range of messages which can be conveyed through physical contact. These 'touch' messages come across with amazing subtlety and tiny nuances, which are perhaps not possible with other methods of communication. What better way to show your feelings for your partner or a good friend than by giving them a caring massage?

The Ultimate Antistress Treatment

The combined benefits of aromatherapy make it the ultimate antistress treatment. But what exactly is stress? The dictionary reads – strain; physical, emotional or mental pressure. Therefore in today's modern world of high pressure and noise we are all under stress to varying degrees every day. Being stressed means remaining in a state of high tension. Too often, many of us are inclined to ignore the warning signs given by our bodies and minds and just keep on going.

But if stress is not controlled it can lead to many symptoms. These can roughly be split into four bands of increasing seriousness. To start with there are the minor symptoms such as tense muscles, headaches, irritability, tiredness and insomnia. Up in the next band, these symptoms operate but as more acute conditions and may develop into muscular pain, chronic aches, persistent infections and mental signs including depression, anxiety, apathy and guilt. If the downward spiral is not halted, it can result in clinical depression, a persecution complex, agoraphobia or claustrophobia and also a susceptibility to infection. In the most serious band of symptoms the body finally begins to collapse with high blood pressure, heart problems, strokes, unexplained pain and an immune system so depressed that it leaves us open to disease.

It makes sense to combat stress as much as possible before it has such drastic and, in the end, life-threatening results. Aromatherapy is a superb antistress and relaxation treatment.

Essential oils and massage work together to relax tense muscles, calm the nervous system and mind, lower the blood pressure and leave the body glowing with a general feeling of well-being. At the same time, aromatherapy is also able to work on the more specific medical symptoms, such as migraine or backache, caused by stress and modern living.

A Complementary Medicine

The modern-day growth of aromatherapy is causing a wealth of lost knowledge and practices to be rediscovered. It was unfortunate that we lost this knowledge before, and it would be equally so to lose that of orthodox and other alternative medicines; because we discover the benefits of one type of medicine, it does not mean that the others have nothing to offer us any more. Therefore the term 'complementary' is carefully chosen. The combined branches of different methods of healing make up the whole tree of medicine.

Viewing medicine in this way also means that a problem can be attacked on more than one front by using different methods of healing. (It is always important to tell your therapist of any other medication you are receiving at the time of treatment.) Although aromatherapy is no substitute for open-heart surgery, its benefits to the body and mind would surely help speed the healing process. A big advantage of aromatherapy is that it does not have the side effects that can occur with conventional medicine, as the essential oils are excreted naturally by the body. Worries about such unwelcome consequences of drugs are nothing new. The British herbalist Culpeper, back in the seventeenth century, wrote passionate denunciations about doctors who used medicines that were poisonous to the body. At the time Culpeper was dismissed as old-fashioned, and despised for clinging to his quaint old herbs, but this thinking is now gaining the backing of modern-day scientific research. His favourite quote, 'The Lord hath created medicines out of the earth, and he that is wise will not abhor them' (Ecclesiasticus 38: 4), neatly illustrates the philosophy that natural is good. Whether or not we attribute her work to God, Mother Nature is a very clever woman. Witness the well-known example of the stinging nettle that grows alongside its antidote – dock leaves.

A further benefit of aromatherapy is that it treats the person with the essential oils that operate in a sensitive and subtle way. Modern-day drugs are designed to cure one single symptom or problem. Essential oils not only treat the specific problem but also help to harmonise and balance the person's mind and body as a whole.

Getting Started – Aromatherapy is Fun!

Aromatherapy is easy and enjoyable. One of its great attributes is that it can be enjoyed in your own home. Do not be put off by the wealth of information and the confusing overlap and numerous properties of the essential oils. There is nothing complicated about a few drops of oil in the bath or giving yourself, or someone else – or even better being given – a massage. Although the recipes are simple to follow, and it is worth doing so for specific reasons and symptoms, do not worry about an exact blend. A good way to explore the properties of oils is to try them individually as bath oils – noticing the effect they have on you. For the more adventurous it is interesting to invent your own blends. As for massage, it does not necessarily require the skills of a trained masseur – oils can turn a humble back-rub into something special. So always follow the dosages laid out and take note of any health warnings – then just have fun!

3
All About Essential Oils

An essential oil is the essence of a single plant. They have also been described as the spirit or soul of a plant. All of us come into regular contact with essential oils, although we may not realise this. We apply essential oils as we put on our favourite perfume or aftershave, as we add herbs, spices or garlic to food, or as we sniff the flowers and plants around us. Essential oils are contained in the tiny oil glands or sacs that surround the flower head and are the most concentrated form of a plant's aromatic materials. The aromas of the plant world are not there simply to perfume the atmosphere, but are highly functional. They attract bees to assist in pollination, repel enemies, and signal to animals whether or not it is safe to eat. The oil of each root, leaf or flower has its own unique fragrance and properties. Even humans have a natural reaction to many smells – we automatically recoil from the smell of sour milk and our own personal aromas have a large part to play in the mating or dating game. An essential oil can be distilled from virtually any plant and there are around 300 of these highly aromatic natural extracts in use by professional aromatherapists today.

Their Nature

Essential oils are not at all like the oils we use for cooking, take on a spoon (such as cod liver oil) or even the oil that we put in the car. In fact, essential oils are chemically distinct and are neither fatty nor greasy. These plant extracts are aromatic, volatile, highly flammable and extremely complex. As we know, essential oils are wonderfully aromatic and each one has its own individual fragrance. Being very volatile means that they evaporate quickly and easily, leaving little or no stain. As for their complexity, essential oils may contain hundreds of different chemical components; as yet, chemists have been unable to reproduce a single one synthetically. Essential oils do not dissolve in water and are generally lighter than water. However they do dissolve in alcohol and mix well with other oils. The majority of essential oils are colourless but some make up a rainbow spectrum of deep reds, browns, blues, greens and yellows.

Extraction

Essential oils are extracted from different parts of the plant depending on the particular oil. For example, jasmine comes from the flowers; tea tree from the leaves and twigs; geranium from the whole plant; sandalwood from the core of the wood itself; and myrrh from a gummy resin. Several different oils may be extracted from different parts of the same species. It usually takes huge amounts of the raw material to produce a small amount of the essential oil. The various growing and picking conditions are also reflected in the price. For example, it takes 60,000 rose blossoms to yield a single ounce of rose oil! Jasmine is another expensive oil as the blooms must be picked by hand before or soon after dawn. By contrast, lavender is much easier to cultivate and the essential oil is far more abundant in the plant. It is therefore cheaper and more widely available. The method of extraction also varies depending upon the plant, although by far the greatest number are extracted by the process of distillation. The various methods of extraction (outlined overleaf) are distillation, enfleurage, expression and solvent extraction.

DISTILLATION

This is a process commonly used in the world of science, but is very useful in the production or purification of many liquids, including alcoholic spirits such as gin or vodka. The use of this process to extract essential oils is an invention generally attributed to the Arabian herbalist, Avicenna, in the eleventh century. During an alchemy experiment using rose petals, he discovered that if the flowers were placed in a flask and heated, the vapour could be collected in another flask. Avicenna identified the fragranced vapour as rosewater and, once condensed, floating on the rosewater's surface was pure rose oil. Today, the modern process operates on exactly the same principle – the aromatic part of the plant is combined with boiling water or steam, the vapour travels along a series of glass tubes that form a condenser and the oil droplets are siphoned off through a narrow-necked container. Gentle prssure or a vacuum can be applied during steam distillation to speed up the process. The possible variation of scale on which this process is carried out is very wide, ranging from small stills beside a field to a large factory. This method is very effective for the extracting of most of the essential oils.

ENFLEURAGE

The oldest method of extraction is in some cases still used, being the best method of obtaining the oil from fragile flower heads such as jasmine. This is because the blossoms continue to release their aroma for twenty-four hours after picking. Within hours of picking, the flowers are placed on sheets of glass that have been covered with purified animal fat or beeswax. As the oil from the flowers soaks into the fat, so more layers of petals are added until the fat is completely saturated with essential oil. The fragrant mulch produced at this stage is called a 'pomade' and at the turn of the century it was used in its raw state as a gentleman's hair dressing. To release the essential oil, the pomade is dissolved in alcohol and the fat sinks to the bottom of the container. The mixture is then heated so that the alcohol evaporates. As enfleurage can only be carried out by hand, it is very much more time consuming than other more mechanised methods. As a result, any essential oil produced in this way is extremely expensive.

EXPRESSION

Citrus oils such as lemon and mandarin are much more readily available as they are found in the multitude of tiny oil glands in the peel of the fruit. You may have noticed this oil squirting out as you peel your fruit. Being so accessible means that the citrus oils can be more easily and cheaply extracted by the method of expression. Originally, the rinds of the fruits were squeezed by hand to extract the oil. Nowadays the process is highly mechanised and the fruit is first crushed before being placed in a centrifugal extractor which rotates at high speed to spin out the droplets of essential oils (exactly the same method as a salad spinner).

SOLVENT EXTRACTION

Technically speaking, this process yields 'absolutes' and not pure essential oils. It is a method primarily used by the perfume industry to release the fragrance from flowers as it is a cheaper alternative to steam distillation. However, for the purposes of aromatherapy the absolutes are not as effective, as the products are devitalised and lacking in therapeutic properties. Solvent extraction is a highly mechanised procedure which begins by mixing flower petals together with a solvent such as hexane in huge metal vats. The mixture is then stirred, encouraging the petals to release their oils. After several hours, the petals are strained off, leaving the solvent and perfumed absolute behind. To retrieve the absolute, the mixture is heated so that the solvent evaporates away. However, some small traces of the solvent inevitably remain in the absolute. Rose, orange blossom and mimosa are the most common absolutes produced by solvent extraction.

How to Buy Essential Oils

A word or two should be said about quality at this point. It is worth bearing in mind that the better the quality of oil you use, the more effective will be the results achieved. First of all it is important to buy only pure essential oil, not one that has been diluted or supplemented. It is also worth looking for essential oils which list the Latin name of the botanic species on the bottle as well as the common name, as the more reputable brands label essential oils with botanical names. Price is also a good indication of quality, but do remember to compare only the same varieties of oil as individual oils vary a great deal in price. As a general rule, you tend to get what you pay for. But do not let this deter you; essential oils are incredibly concentrated so you will only need a few drops at a time. The aroma itself is also an indication of a quality essential oil. The scent of a good quality oil has a brilliance and vitality lacking in their poorer counterparts. If you place a good essential oil on the table in front of you and remove the lid, you should be able to smell the aroma without bringing it any closer to your nose. The scent of a poor quality oil will not rise up in the same way.

Do not worry if the fragrance of any essential oil varies from year to year, or batch to batch. This is inevitable as they are like fine wines and vary with the area, the year, the weather, the picking conditions and so on. In fact, if the smell remains constant year after year it is a good indication that the oil has been tampered with or was produced artificially. Also, keep in mind that essential oils are a natural product. This means that there are no definite rules which divide the good oils from the bad ones, but rather a complete spectrum of different quality oils. As with buying fruit, there are many different classes and the price you pay depends on the quality you buy.

Despite the vast number of different essential oils on the market, you only need buy a few to get started. A handful of those mentioned in the following A–Z and one or two of the carrier oils will be plenty for a beginner. As you experiment, so your collection of small bottles will expand. I recommend the following seven essential oils as a starter kit for a good, basic aromatherapy cabinet:

Chamomile
Eucalyptus
Geranium
Lavender
Rosewood
Tangerine
Ylang ylang

Stored correctly, essential oils will last several years. The exceptions are the citrus oils which should be used within one year of opening. However, all essential oils are affected by heat, light, air and plastic. Follow these three golden rules to keep your essential oils in tip-top condition for at least six months:

* Store in glass bottles with the tops firmly closed. Screw caps are better than cork-stoppers.
* All oil bottles should be dark in colour and the best are amber or dark blue. Good quality essential oils are always sold in coloured glass.
* Keep bottles in a cool place, such as a cupboard, away from sunlight or a radiator.

——4——
The A-Z of Essential Oils

All essential oils are antiseptic to varying degrees. Many are far more powerful than phenol which is the active ingredient in most commercial cleansing materials. However, they are far kinder on the skin and smell much more pleasant! The essential oils are so effective because of their antibiotic, antibacterial and antiviral properties – they attack germs without damaging the body. Some of them also help to heal and maintain health by stimulating and boosting the body's own immune system, cardiovascular supply and the lymphatic defences. Not only do essential oils have these and other medicinal properties, but they can also have a profound effect on the mind and the emotions. They may play an important part in our mental health, or on a smaller scale they may alter our mood of the moment. Some essential oils such as lavender even seem to have a balancing action, acting as a sedative or tonic depending on the state of the person concerned.

There are several hundred essential oils that come from all corners of the world. In this *Quick Guide*, I will concentrate on those most commonly available and most interesting for everyday use. These are outlined in the A–Z listing below. Essential oils are complex, so the description of each oil may not be exhaustive. However, it is important not to be daunted by each oil's range of properties, or the frequent overlap of functions. That versatility is one of the major beauties of the essential oils. If more than one oil fits your need – look at their other properties, blend some together – or simply pick the aroma you prefer. Prices vary enormously. At the lower end of the scale (inexpensive) expect to pay £3–£4. For the more expensive oils, expect to pay £20–£40 for a small bottle.

BASIL *(Ocimum basilicum)*

The name comes from the Greek basileús, meaning king. This small aromatic bush with white flowers has been cultivated in Europe since the twelfth century. In India it is traditionally revered as sacred, being dedicated to the Hindu gods Krishna and Vishnu. Worldwide there are over 150 varieties of basil. The oil is distilled from the leaves and flowering tops of the herb.

Description: Revitalising, smelling slightly of camphor.

Uses: A natural tranquilliser with a mentally stimulating effect which helps in conditions of stress and fights fatigue. Burning a few drops in a diffuser encourages mental concentration. Good in massage blends, having a toning effect on the skin and being useful in the treatment of cellulite. It is used by aromatherapists to help ease the digestive tract and regulate the menstrual cycle.

Price: Moderate cost.

Safety: A powerful oil that should not be used during pregnancy or on children. An excess can act as a depressant.

BAY *(Laurus nobilis)*

Bay trees grow wild in the West Indies. Their leaves have a pungent taste and aroma and are often used in cooking. The essential oil is stored in tiny glands on the surface of the leaves which release a delicious scent when pressed or shaken. This fragrance made the bay especially popular with the Romans who gave bay-leaf garlands to their army and literary heroes.

Description: Uplifting with a warm, spicy smell.

Uses: A good all-round tonic – makes a fortifying bath oil. Useful for treating respiratory disorders, depression and aches, sprains and rheumatism. Add to scalp oils to discourage hair loss and treat dandruff.

Price: Relatively inexpensive.

Bergamot *(Citrus bergamia)*

Named after the Italian town of Bergamo where the fruit was originally cultivated. Bergamot oil is pressed from the oil-bearing glands on the surface of the fruit, which is a cross between an orange and a lemon. It is used to flavour Earl Grey tea and is a traditional ingredient in eau-de-Cologne.

Description: A deliciously fresh aroma smelling of sweet oranges.

Uses: The treatment of infected skin conditions such as boils, spots and ulcers. Aromatherapists use it to help combat intestinal problems and infections of the urinary tract. Add to massage blends for beating depression as its attractive aroma can improve mood and help focus the mind. Suits combination and oily skin types.

Price: Moderate cost.

Safety: Citrus oils react to sunlight and should not be used on the skin while sunbathing or before using a sun-bed.

Cajuput *(Melaleuca minor)*

Also called the swamp tea tree, this Indonesian tree has small fragrant white flowers that cluster around a long spike. The source of the essential oil is the leaves, twigs and fresh buds of the tree.

Description: A strong, clear smell similar to rosemary.

Uses: Improves mood and increases resistance to infections, especially coughs, colds and 'flu. Add to massage blends, bath oils or use as a purifying room fragrance. Aromatherapists use in the treatment of gynaecological problems including painful periods and cystitis.

Price: Inexpensive.

Cedarwood *(Cedrus atlantica)*

The oil has been in use for thousands of years and was burnt in Ancient Egyptian and Greek temples as incense. The temple of

Solomon in Jerusalem was built entirely of cedarwood and the amount used was so great that the forests of Lebanon have never fully recovered. Burning cedarwood chippings on the fire is a delightfully subtle way of scenting a room. Today, the oil is extracted from sawdust and wood shavings saved from American cedar mills – very environmentally friendly!

Description: A harmonious, woody smell.

Uses: Treatment of respiratory disorders including bronchitis and catarrh. May relieve aching muscles and helps firm and tone the skin. Suits oily and combination skin and may be added to jojoba oil to treat acne. Can give a calming influence and helps focus the mind. A meditative room fragrance.

Price: Inexpensive.

CHAMOMILE *(Athemia nobilis)*

A common plant in temperate regions all over Europe and is named after the Greek for 'ground apple' due to the apple-like scent it releases when trodden on. Chamomile (or camomile) is traditionally associated with the nobility and the lawns at Buckingham Palace are laid with this herb. A blue or pale yellow oil is produced from the dried flowers.

Description: A gentle oil with a warm, fruity aroma.

Uses: This versatile oil belongs in the first-aid box as it can be used to treat nerves, headaches, insomnia and menstrual disorders. Also useful for skin complaints as it is one of the few essential oils that can be applied to inflamed skin conditions. Add to facial massage oils to soothe dry, oily or irritated skin conditions. Especially recommended for babies and children – it is wonderful in the bath to encourage a good night's sleep.

Price: Relatively expensive.

CLARY SAGE *(Salvia sclarea)*

Clary sage is native to Spain. This attractive plant with large purple flowers and pineapple-scented leaves is traditionally associated with feminine sexuality and gynaecology. The oil is distilled from the flowering tops and leaves.

Description: A slightly sour, nutty aroma that can be quite powerful.

Uses: Contains a hormone-like compound similar to oestrogen that is reputed to regulate hormonal imbalance so is excellent in the treatment of pre-menstrual syndrome and symptoms of the menopause. A good way to utilise this is through massage. Inhaling or using the oil in the bath can help lift post-natal depression. It is good as a general room essence to improve mood and mental clarity.

Price: Medium cost.

Safety: Avoid during pregnancy.

CYPRESS *(Cupressus sempervirens)*

This large evergreen tree is common in southern Europe. The first recorded use of cypress oil was about 2,000 years ago, when a Greek physician named Dioscorides claimed it to be a cure for diarrhoea. The ancient oil is extracted from the needles and twigs of the tree.

Description: A refreshing smell similar to pine needles.

Uses: Increases the circulation and works as a gentle treatment for water retention. Useful for menopausal problems, stress and nervous tension. Good in body massage blends to improve skin tone, encourage the elimination of toxins and help the condition of cellulite. Being mildly astringent it is better for oily and combination skins. For sweaty feet cypress makes an excellent footbath. A very good burning essence, especially for invalids and hospital wards.

Price: Moderate cost.

EUCALYPTUS *(Eucalyptus smithii)*

Native to Australia, eucalyptus shoots are the favourite food of the koala. There are many different varieties but only fifteen of them are used to make essential oils, which come from the leaves and older branches. Eucalyptus is one of the most important essential oils used in pharmacy.

Description: Vigorous with a clear, powerful aroma.

Uses: It helps clear the respiratory tract and is useful in treating sinusitis and head colds, so it makes a purifying burning essence, or an invigorating steam inhalation. It may also help to ease migraine. Use in massage to help reduce the pain of rheumatism and arthritis. One drop in jojoba oil is a useful treatment for acne and spotty complexions.

Price: Inexpensive.

Safety: A powerful oil to be used sparingly.

FRANKINCENSE *(Boswellia carterii)*

The essential oil is found in the gummy resin given out by the bark of the tree, which is native to Somalia. The name comes from the mediaeval French. Frankincense has been a symbol of divinity for thousands of years and was one of the gifts bought by the three kings for the infant Christ.

Description: A lightly spiced, slightly camphoric smell.

Uses: The pungent aroma helps focus the mind and this oil has meditative qualities. It is also good for the treatment of stress and nervous tension. A useful oil to burn when overworked or trying to cope under pressure, or alternatively a few drops rubbed into the scalp helps clear the mind and encourage mental stimulation. Used in facial oils to deter fine lines and wrinkles.

Price: Fairly expensive.

GERANIUM *(Pelargonium graveolens)*

There are over 700 different types of geranium flower but only seven are used to make essential oils. The oil is extracted from the whole plant, which is gathered before flowering. The strongest scented is called Geranium Bourbon and comes from the Ile de Réunion in the Indian Ocean. This is an important ingredient in Estée Lauder's famous 'Youth Dew' perfume.

Description: A sweet, rose-like aroma.

Uses: One of the most useful oils as it suits all skin types including dry, oily and sensitive. Soothes skin irritations and is particularly effective in the treatment of problem skin. Also helps to heal burns and minor abrasions. Due to these properties and lovely smell it is an excellent addition to massage oils. Geranium is used by aromatherapists for a wide range of ailments including hormonal and menstrual problems. It is worth noting that this oil is safe for diluted external use during pregnancy.

Price: Relatively inexpensive.

HYSSOP *(Hyssopus officinalis)*

A flowering herb native to Europe, hyssop is also widely cultivated in Brazil and the Middle East. The highly fragrant oil, found in the leaves, is an important ingredient for the perfume-making industry.

Description: A spicy scent similar to thyme or basil.

Uses: Treatment of respiratory infections including coughs, colds and 'flu. Promotes the healing of bruised skin and is useful in combating the aches of rheumatism and arthritis – use in compresses on bruised or aching limbs. Add to facial massage blends to treat dry and sensitive complexions. If burned as a room fragrance, hyssop gives off a warm, vibrant aroma.

Price: Relatively expensive.

Safety: A powerful oil to be used sparingly and not at all during pregnancy.

JASMINE *(Jasminum officinale)*

Jasmine oil is one of the most expensive essential oils as a vast number of flowers are needed to make a tiny amount of the oil. Labour costs are made high as the blossoms have to be picked before or soon after dawn due to changes in the plant's internal chemistry. The oil is still occasionally extracted by enfleurage from the pink jasmine flowers. Once extracted, the oil later develops into a rich shade of ruby red. A very important ingredient for the perfume industry as it is the heart of many fine fragrances, including 'Chanel No. 5', 'Samsara' by Guerlain and 'Anaïs Anaïs' by Cacharel. The highest quality jasmine oil comes from Grasse in the south of France, where it has been grown for hundreds of years.

Description: Uplifting with an exquisitely heady, floral fragrance.

Uses: Will invigorate and lift depression and is calming to the nervous system. Used to treat menstrual disorders, stress and general anxiety. Although expensive it only needs to be used in tiny quantities. One or two drops make a luxurious bath oil or an excellent addition to massage oils for the face and body. Reputed to repair skin tissues and can be used in small quantities during pregnancy to help prevent stretch marks. Suits all skin types, especially the sensitive and dry.

Price: Extremely expensive. Ylang ylang is sometimes used as a less expensive alternative.

JUNIPER BERRY *(Juniperus communis)*

Juniper is a small, grey-green leafed bush which grows in many regions of the world, including central and southern Europe, North America and Canada. Juniper berries are used to give gin its distinctive, bitter flavour. The oil is distilled from the ripe, dried berries.

Description: A pungent, woody smell.

Uses: A medicinal oil that is used by aromatherapists to treat digestive, urinary and hormonal problems. Also used by practitioners to treat liver problems and combat chronic obesity. Good for treating problem skins and a few drops can be used in facial oils for treating acne. It is also suitable for oily and combination skins. Add a few drops to a bath to relieve tired, aching limbs or use in a massage to combat cellulite.

Price: Moderate cost.

Safety: Avoid during pregnancy.

LAVENDER *(Lavendula officinalis)*

From the Latin *lavare* meaning 'to wash', lavender has been used for centuries for skin care and in fragrances. The oil was the first British essential oil to be distilled commercially in the late seventeenth century and is the main ingredient in lavender water which was created at about the same time. The source of the oil is the tiny green pods that sit either side of the pale purple flowers.

Description: Balancing with a delicate and well-loved fragrance.

Uses: Probably the most useful of all essential oils and a *must* for the first-aid box. Apply neat to heal burns and dilute with wheat-germ oil to repair scar tissue. Also used by aromatherapists to treat abrasions, coughs, colds, 'flu, stress, nausea, ulcers, acne, boils, asthma and rheumatism. Helps relieve headaches and migraines. Lavender has an amazing balancing action and either calms or stimulates according to the body needs, generally producing a state of well-being. It is very useful for massage, in the bath and as a room fragrancer. Suits most skin types except the very dry.

Price: Inexpensive.

LEMON *(Citrus limonum)*

Lemon oil is one of the easiest oils to extract from the oil glands on the fruit's outer peel. It is a traditional antiseptic and purifier. Associated with the hair and scalp, it is reputed to stimulate hair growth and will bleach the hair blonde if applied prior to exposure to the sun.

Description: Stimulating with a sharp, refreshing smell.

Uses: Strengthens the immune system and helps ward off infections. Also useful to treat colds, sinusitis and sore throats. It can be used neat in small quantities as an antiseptic. Aromatherapists treat digestive disorders, gallstones, fever and anxiety with lemon essential oil. Add to massage oils to help improve blood circulation, tone flabby skin and help combat cellulite. It can also be burned in an oil burner as an insect repellent.

Price: Very inexpensive. Citrus oils should be used within one year of purchase.

Safety: Citrus oils react strongly to sunlight and should not be used on the skin while sunbathing or before using a sun-bed.

MANDARIN (*Citrus deliciosa*)

Originally native to Italy, this fruit is an important crop in Italy, Brazil, Spain, Argentina and China. An inexpensive oil, it is an important ingredient in cheaper fragrances. As with all the citrus fruits, the oil is stored in the tiny glands on the peel.

Description: Full of zest!

Uses: A general tonic and natural tranquilliser, which can help with insomnia, stress and nervous tension – add to a warm bath for an uplifting effect. During pregnancy use in massage oils to boost the circulation and discourage water retention. Good for combination and problem skins.

Price: Inexpensive. Citrus oils should be used within one year of purchase.

Safety: Citrus oils react strongly to sunlight and should not be used on the skin while sunbathing or before using a sun-bed.

MARJORAM (*Origanum majorana*)

This herb is native to Hungary. In hot climates the plant secretes a sweet, sticky resin from its stems which is popular with honey bees. The oil is extracted from the flowering tops and leaves.

Description: Comforting with a warm, spicy aroma.

Uses: Regulates the nervous system and induces drowsiness, so is used to treat insomnia. Try a few drops in the bath before bedtime. Used by aromatherapists to treat menstrual problems, menopausal disorders, anxiety and stress. May also help to ease intestinal cramps. Add to massage oils to treat strained muscles and tired, aching limbs. Suits oily and combination complexions.

Price: Fairly expensive.

Safety: Avoid during pregnancy.

MELISSA *(Melissa officinalis)*

Melissa thrives in Mediterranean countries and is also known as **lemon balm** as the leaves release a lemon-like fragrance when pressed between the palms. This highly prized fragrance was the world's first unisex scent, worn by both noblemen and women.

Description: A subtle herby aroma with a touch of lemon.

Uses: Can help treat nerves, overexertion, jet lag and stress. Use in the bath to unwind and promote relaxation, or add to reviving massage blends for use after exercise. Useful against digestive and bacterial disorders. Suits all skin types.

Price: Pure melissa oil is both rare and extremely expensive. Most liquids sold as melissa oil are a much cheaper blend of citrus oils.

MYRRH *(Commiphora myrrha)*

Myrrh is a small, thorny bush growing in north-east Africa and Arabia. One of the oldest known perfumes, it was used by the Ancient Egyptians in the embalming process and to perfume linen. Myrrh was highly valued and was brought as a gift by one of the three kings for the infant Christ. Medicinally myrrh has been associated traditionally with the mouth. Distillation of the resin (crude myrrh) produces the pure essential oil.

Description: A rich, spicy and slightly musty aroma.

Uses: Treatment of chronic chest complaints such as bronchitis and catarrh. Improves digestive disorders and is used in the treatment of fungal infections, including candidiasis. Helps heal burns and minor skin abrasions and is popular in skin-care oils to soothe angry, inflamed skin. Add a few drops to face and body massage oils to strengthen and tone the skin. Suits combination and problem skins.

Price: Relatively expensive.

Safety: Avoid during pregnancy.

NEROLI *(Citrus aurantium)*

Named after Flavio Orsini, Prince of Nerola in the sixteenth century, whose wife loved the flower's heady fragrance, the essential oil is taken from the flowers of the bitter orange and is also known as orange blossom or orange flower oil. It remains an important ingredient in modern eau-de-Colognes.

Description: Warming with a distinctively soft, fruity and refreshing aroma.

Uses: The perfume creates a warm and relaxing atmosphere, making a wonderful and fragrant bath. It is excellent for relieving anxiety and nervous tension, calming pre-exam or interview nerves and is used to treat stage fright. Useful for menopausal and hormonal disorders. In a massage oil it can help improve a sluggish circulation and tired complexion. Also used in blends to treat problem skins and acne (suits oilier skin types).

Price: Very expensive.

PATCHOULI *(Pogostemon patchouli)*

Found in the Far East and the West Indies, this plant looks similar to melissa (lemon balm). The dried leaves of the herb produce a rich, claret-coloured oil with legendary skin-care attributes. The first recorded use of patchouli oil in Europe was by the weavers of Paisley in Scotland who discovered that they could not compete with the Indian shawl exporters unless they impregnated their cloth with the same fragrance.

Description: Soothing with a heavy, Indian aroma.

Uses: Calms fevers and inflamed skin conditions. It is especially good when diluted with wheat-germ oil to soothe burns and scar tissue. Helps treat fungal infections, acne and scalp disorders including dryness and dandruff, so it is a useful addition to skin-care and scalp oils. Suits most complexions and skin types. Gives off an attractive, heady aroma when burned and a few drops in the bath water turn bathing into a sensual treat.

Price: Inexpensive.

PEPPERMINT *(Mentha piperita)*

This European herb was named by the British botanist John Rea in 1700 for its peppery smell. Peppermint leaves contain the compound menthol which contributes to its strong smell and feeling of coldness when rubbed onto the skin. The essential oil is traditionally used in aftershaves and skin tonics for its invigorating and bracing action.

Description: Cooling with a strong, fresh smell.

Uses: Clears the head and encourages positive thinking. It is used to treat headaches, migraine and insomnia. Add to massage oils for its invigorating and refreshing effect. Has an antispasmodic action useful for relieving wind, heartburn, indigestion, nausea and colic. Not a good bath oil as it can make the water feel cold against the skin; however it does make a wonderfully refreshing foot bath.

Price: Very inexpensive. Tends not to keep for more than one year.

PETITGRAIN *(Citrus aurantium)*

This oil comes from the leaves and twigs of the orange tree, traditionally grown in the warm, humid climates of southern France, Morocco and West Africa. The name petitgrain comes from the French for 'little bit', referring to the tiny droplets of oil encapsulated in the leaves.

Description: A woody, floral aroma.

Uses: Treatment of an overburdened nervous system and relief of anxiety and tension. A good general aid to convalescence as it gives off a warm, heartening aroma when burned. Useful for insomnia and a few drops added to a bath before bedtime promotes sleep. An excellent oil to add to massage blends.

Price: Inexpensive.

PINE *(Pinus palustris)*

One of the first essential oils documented by Dr Jean Valnet for its power to prevent respiratory disorders. Pine essential oil is associated with cleanliness and freshness and is commonly added to medicated soaps and household cleaners. It is extracted from the needles and twigs from the tree.

Description: A strong, fresh, forest smell.

Uses: Treatment of colds, 'flu, bronchitis and other respiratory infections. A few drops in a bowl of hot water makes a steam inhalation. Strongly antiseptic, making it good for general infections and minor skin abrasions. One or two drops in the bath will help stave off infections and boost a sluggish circulation. Alternatively it can be burned to give off a cleansing aroma. Used by aromatherapists to help with bladder and kidney disorders and to improve the circulation.

Price: Inexpensive.

Safety: A potent oil which should be used sparingly and avoided during pregnancy.

ROSE OTTO *(Rosa damascena)*

A beautiful flowering plant that originated in Persia and has since been introduced to all temperate regions. The true rose essential oil, rose otto, comes from the ruby-red damask rose petals. Legend has it that these were created from a single drop of sweat falling from Mohammad's brow. The flower later gave its name to the city of Damascus and the heavy silk fabric that was originally woven there. Pure rose oil contains over 500 different chemical constituents and so far has proved impossible for the cosmetic chemists to copy exactly. Despite its expense rose oil remains one of the most important perfume ingredients and rose otto is found in many fine fragrances including 'Chanel No. 5', Estée Lauder's 'White Linen' and 'Fidji' by Guy Laroche.

Description: Uplifting with a wonderful, warm, floral fragrance.

Uses: Useful to treat mild depression and fatigue. Rose essential oil can help pre-menstrual syndrome and symptoms of the menopause. Suits and soothes dry, mature and sensitive skins. A luxury oil to be used sparingly in facial massage blends or

added in tiny quantities to a bath. A wonderful oil for children and fabulous for pampering the body during pregnancy.
Price: Very expensive.

ROSE ABSOLUTE *(Rosa centifolia)* is widely used in aromatherapy although it is not a true essential oil. It is also commonly used in sweetmeats such as Turkish delight. It is produced by solvent extraction from the pale pink centifolia rose and, unfortunately, traces of the chemical solvent may be carried through to the end product. What is sold is likely to be a dilution of the absolute as pure rose absolute is highly concentrated and expensive. Although rose absolute is a cheaper alternative to rose otto and often used in skin care, it is still expensive. Similar scents are rose geranium and rosewood.

ROSEMARY *(Rosmarinus officinalis)*

A shrubby bush found in many Mediterranean countries and the former Soviet Union. It was regarded as a sacred herb by the Ancient Greeks and Romans, and often used in their rituals. Rosemary oil, from the herb's flowering tops, was also the base for the world's first commercially produced perfume called Hungary water, formulated by Italian monks in 1370.
Description: An invigorating spicy aroma.
Uses: An excellent all-round tonic. Helps combat water retention and cellulite, tones flabby skin, and may combat dandruff and hair loss. Suits problem skins and oilier complexions. Has pain-relieving properties so is useful to treat headaches, aching limbs and to heal sprains. It may also help rheumatism and arthritis.
Price: Inexpensive.
Safety: An excess can induce epilepsy in predisposed persons. Avoid during pregnancy.

ROSEWOOD *(Aniba rosaeodora)*

This oil is distilled from the bark of a tall South American tree, called rosewood after its lightly rose-scented wood. The essential oil is also known by the more romantic name of Bois de Rose and can be used as a cheaper alternative to the genuine rose petal oils, although it has fewer therapeutic benefits. Rosewood tends to be from unsustainable forests and may not therefore be an environmentally sound choice.

Description: Refreshing with a mellow, floral aroma.

Uses: A gentle tonic, which works well as an antidepressant or general mood improver. It makes for a good pick-me-up in the bath. Relieves headaches and may help with migraines. Use instead of rose for its scent, but remember it has far reduced skin-care properties by comparison.

Price: Moderate cost.

SAGE *(Salvia officinalis)*

Sage was a sacred herb in ancient times. An important ingredient in Chinese herbal medicine, it grows almost anywhere but predominantly in Mediterranean countries. The essential oil is distilled from the flowers and leaves.

Description: A pungent, herbaceous smell.

Uses: A useful regulator of the central nervous system. Aromatherapists may use sage to treat depression, and severe menstrual and digestive disorders. Useful against catarrh, bronchitis and other chest conditions.

Price: Moderate cost.

Safety: A powerful oil which can easily overstimulate. Use only under the guidance of an aromatherapist and not at all during pregnancy.

SANDALWOOD *(Santalum album)*

A traditional Indian extract, this essential oil comes from a parasitic tree that grows by attaching its roots to others. Much used by Hindus in temples and at religious occasions; for example, as a paste on the forehead it is a symbol of purity for spiritual leaders. It is one of the slowest growing trees and it takes forty years before the essential oil can be extracted, from sawdust and wood chippings. The wood itself is popular for furniture making as it resists attack from pests, notably woodworm.

Description: Gentle with a rich and comforting aroma.

Uses: Induces calm and a sense of well-being. A few drops make a lovely pick-me-up in the bath. Helps with pre-menstrual syndrome and is reputed to strengthen the immune system. Also used by aromatherapists to treat impotence. Can be added to massage blends to treat sore, inflamed skin conditions. Suits irritated, flaky complexions and is useful in facial oil blends for blemishes and acne.

Price: Fairly expensive.

TANGERINE *(Citrus nobilis)*

Tangerine trees come from the same botanical source as mandarin, therefore their essential oils are chemically very similar. As with all the citrus fruits the essential oil is extracted by expression from the peel.

Description: Uplifting, with a fresh, tangy aroma.

Uses: This cheering essential oil is a natural tonic. Can help in cases of depression and is excellent in morning baths. This all-rounder alleviates aches and pains, cellulite and disorders of the digestive system. Especially useful in massage oils for the pregnant as it gently stimulates the circulation.

Price: Inexpensive.

Safety: Citrus oils react strongly to sunlight and should not be used on the skin while sunbathing or before using a sun-bed. Citrus oils should be used within one year of purchase.

TEA TREE *(Melaleuca alternifolia)*

This is a common Australian tree which is extremely resistant to disease. It also has amazing powers of recuperation and if chopped down will quickly grow again from its original stump. Originally the oil was used in aboriginal medicine, but it is now also being used increasingly by conventional medics. Tea tree oil is five times more effective at killing germs than household disinfectant, while also being far kinder to the skin. The essential oil is distilled from the leaves and twigs.

Description: A pungent, medicinal smell.

Uses: Very useful against fungal conditions such as candida and bacterial infections. Can help ward off coughs, colds and 'flu. Also useful for the treatment of skin disorders including cold sores, warts, burns and acne. Use neat in very small amounts to treat spots, burns and insect bites. Add to scalp oils to treat dandruff and scalp disorders. A few drops in the bath can combat the effects of shock and hysteria.

Price: Inexpensive.

THYME *(Thymus vulgaris)*

One of the most widely used herbs in herbal medicine throughout history. Traditionally burned as a household disinfectant to ward off rodents and get rid of fleas. Sachets of dried thyme or handkerchiefs sprinkled with essential oil can be hung in wardrobes instead of moth-balls. The oil is obtained from the flowering tops of the herb.

Description: Stimulating with a sharp, herby smell.

Uses: A strong antiseptic, it is used by aromatherapists as a general tonic to relieve fatigue and anxiety. It is also useful for relieving tired, aching limbs. Stimulates the circulation and encourages the elimination of toxins. Thyme essential oil can lower blood pressure and regulate the menstrual cycle. Reputed to strengthen the immune system. Dilute and massage into the neck for an effective remedy to treat sore throats and tonsillitis.

Price: Inexpensive.
Safety: A powerful oil that should only be used under the guidance of an aromatherapist and not at all during pregnancy.

YLANG YLANG *(Cananga odorata)*

An attractive, flowering tree originally grown in Indonesia but now cultivated in the Comoro Islands, north-west of Madagascar. Its flowers are bright yellow and have long flowing petals. The name ylang ylang comes from the Malay for 'flower of flowers'. The essential oil is extracted from freshly picked flower petals.

Description: An exotic, heady fragrance similar to jasmine.
Uses: Regulates the nervous system and lowers blood pressure. Useful during times of depression, stress and overwork – burning the oil helps to combat these. A few drops also create a reviving bath. Some aromatherapists may use it as a treatment for impotence and frigidity.
Price: Medium cost. Can be used as a less expensive alternative to jasmine.
Safety: An excess may cause headaches. Use with caution in massage blends as it can occasionally provoke an allergic reaction.

——— 5 ———
Aromatherapy in Practice

Carrier Oils

For massage and most direct application to the skin, the essential oils must always be mixed with a carrier oil (for the recommended dilutions see page 49–50). This is because essential oils are too highly concentrated to use neat on the skin. There are just a few specific exceptions, such as lavender oil on burns and small cuts, and tea tree oil on spots and warts (in these cases only tiny amounts, one or two drops should be used). Any other direct application of neat essential oils should only be undertaken by a trained aromatherapist.

The carrier or base oils used to dilute essential oils come from vegetables, nuts or seeds. Readily absorbed by the skin, many of them have therapeutic properties of their own and it is important to buy unrefined, cold-pressed oils to gain the full benefit of these. The oils outlined below are safe for all skin types, but it may be worthwhile carrying out a patch test with the carrier oils you intend to use, as a few people may have a reaction even to natural oils. To conduct a patch test, simply apply the oil to a small area, such as the inner arm, and wait to see if there is any adverse reaction over the following twenty-four hours. When making your own recipes, it is also a good idea to use a blend of base oils to get the most from their various benefits. This is also a cheaper alternative to using a single, expensive carrier oil.

The most common carrier (or base) oils are listed here.

ALMOND OIL

This is sweet almond oil (bitter almond oil is not sold as it is highly toxic and contains cyanide). It is a slightly sticky oil especially suited to body massage blends. Good for most skin types particularly dry, easily irritated complexions. It can help relieve itching and soreness. Rich in skin nourishing nutrients, it is a versatile oil.

APRICOT-KERNEL OIL

The light texture of this oil is especially suitable for facial blends. Mature, dry, sensitive or inflamed skins benefit from its natural store of vitamins and minerals. An expensive oil to use on its own, it works well when blended with less costly almond, grapeseed or jojoba oils.

AVOCADO OIL

One of the richest carrier oils, it is useful for treating mature and dehydrated skins, and can also help relieve eczema and psoriasis. It contains protein, vitamins (especially vitamin E), lecithin and essential fatty acids. This oil is good as an enriching addition to a blend of other carrier oils, using up to approximately one-tenth of the final mixture.

BORAGE OIL

A nourishing oil which is useful in the treatment of skin disorders such as eczema and psoriasis. Due to its essential fatty acid content, borage oil may also be an effective anti-ageing treatment. This oil is best used as an addition to a blend as it is very expensive. The easiest way is to pierce a capsule and add the contents to your mixture.

CAMELLIA OIL

A Japanese oil which is readily absorbed to soften and smooth the skin. Suited to all skin types it is a good addition to massage blends. Traditionally camellia oil is also used in hair care, including conditioning treatments.

Carrot Oil
An excellent source of vitamins, especially beta-carotene, it may be used to help heal scar tissue. Suited to facial oils to combat acne and irritated skin. Use well diluted as an excess can stain the skin yellow.

Evening Primrose Oil
Containing the nutrients gamma linoleic acid (GLA), vitamins and minerals, this oil combats dry, devitalised skin, eczema and may even help to prevent premature skin ageing. As with borage oil, the easiest way to use this expensive liquid is by adding the contents of a capsule to your blend. Liquid evening primrose oil is often poor quality. The capsules are a better bet as they comply with strict pharmaceutical standards.

Grapeseed Oil
A favourite with aromatherapists for its light texture and lack of smell. The oil is non-greasy and excellent for body massage blends. It suits all skin types, but is not a particularly nourishing oil so benefits from the addition of other oils. However, it is also perfectly acceptable on its own. This all-rounder has other important attributes – it is inexpensive and can be found in most supermarkets.

Hazelnut Oil
This oil is extremely light and so suits oily or combination skins. Very easily absorbed it is excellent for face and massage blends. Being relatively costly, it is a good combination with grapeseed or sunflower oils.

Jojoba Oil

Pronounced 'ho-ho-ba', jojoba oil is a wonderfully light carrier oil and is the best base for facial oil blends. It also works well as a body oil and penetrates the skin easily. Its composition is similar to sebum, the skin's natural oil produced by the sebaceous glands. It suits all skin types but especially oily, combination and acne-prone skins. Jojoba oil is often used in skin- and hair-care products.

Kiwi-seed Oil

A nourishing oil which is imported from New Zealand. This pale yellow oil is a useful skin conditioner, as it contains a good level of essential fatty acids to encourage cell renewal and improve general skin tone. A light oil which is especially good in body massage blends.

Kukui-nut Oil

This oil has in the past been used as a holy anointing oil. Today, its many useful characteristics are known and utilised. The oil penetrates deep into the layers of the skin, carrying essential fatty acids. Kukui-nut oil is soothing and healing in cases of sunburn, skin irritation or chapped skin. This gentle caring oil makes an ideal baby-care oil.

Macadamia-nut Oil

This oil has a wonderful silky texture and is quickly absorbed into the skin, so it is useful for both facial and body massage blends. Due to its particular fatty acid composition, macadamia-nut oil helps to protect skin cells and is a lovely oil to use on more mature skins.

Olive Oil

This common cooking oil is conveniently available in its cold-pressed, unrefined state from most supermarkets. As a carrier oil it does however have a very distinctive smell which is not everyone's cup of tea. Bottles labelled 'pure' olive oil are more refined and deodorised to remove the smell. Its slightly sticky texture suits dryer skins. Very good for body massage blends and for soothing sore, dehydrated or chapped skin.

PASSIONFLOWER OIL

A nourishing oil which helps maintain skin elasticity, it is an excellent addition to face and body massage blends. It also has mild anti-inflammatory properties and so is very useful when treating irritated skin. The easiest way to use passionflower oil is to pierce a capsule and add the contents to enrich your blend.

PEACH-NUT OIL

A useful source of essential fatty acids, vitamins and minerals. Peach-nut oil is a very good addition to face and body massage blends. It helps prevent skin dehydration and is especially suitable for the more sensitive complexions.

ROSE-HIP OIL

A superbly textured carrier oil. Having a higher therapeutic activity than any other carrier oil, rose-hip oil is extremely useful to help the healing of scars and skin burns. It may also be of use in blends for prematurely ageing skin. However it is very expensive and for the majority of us, evening primrose is probably a more viable alternative. Rose-hip oil is also known as muscat oil and is sold by some professional aromatherapy suppliers.

SAFFLOWER OIL

Another favourite with aromatherapists for body massage because of its light texture and penetrative power. It suits all skin types and unrefined versions contain useful amounts of vitamins (especially E) and minerals. Safflower oil is also one of the cheapest and most readily available oils.

SESAME OIL

A nourishing oil containing vitamins, minerals and the essential fatty acid lecithin. Plain, untoasted sesame oil can be used to help skin complaints such as eczema and psoriasis. Suiting all skin types it is an excellent addition to facial oils, using about one-tenth of the final blend.

SUNFLOWER OIL

Inexpensive and light in texture, this oil is especially good for body massage. It suits all skin types and blends well with the more exotic oils. Make sure you use an unrefined variety as most are highly processed and likely to contain traces of solvents. Unrefined sunflower oil is also a good source of natural vitamin E.

WALNUT OIL

Walnuts themselves taste delicious and walnut oil can also be used in the kitchen adding a very distinctive flavour to a whole range of dishes. In the role of a carrier oil it is nourishing as it is high in essential fatty acids. Easily absorbed with a smooth texture, walnut oil is best added to body massage blends.

WHEATGERM OIL

This dark, aromatic oil is too sticky to use on its own but makes a wonderful addition to dry skin massage blends. Wheatgerm oil is our best source of vitamin E, so it is especially good for healing scar tissue and burns. Add a few drops from a capsule to every massage blend as it is a natural antioxidant and will help to preserve the oils and prevent rancidity.

Note: People with a wheat allergy may be sensitive to this oil so you should carry out a patch test before using. If there is a reaction, avocado oil is an alternative source of vitamin E, although not as potent.

Massage

The mainstay of aromatherapy, massage is a wonderful way of utilising the essential oils.

Blending your oil
Pick your carrier oils, place in a glass bottle and shake well. Add the drops of your chosen essential oils, taking care not to exceed the recommended dosage, and shake well again.

Dosage
* *Adults:* One drop of essential oil to 1ml of carrier oil, i.e. five drops to every 5ml, ten drops to every 10ml and so on. It is useful to know that 5ml = 1 teaspoon, 10ml = 1 dessertspoon and 15ml = 1 tablespoon.
* *Children aged 1–3 months:* use under a quarter the above strength.
* *Children aged 3–18 months:* use a quarter the strength.
* *Children aged 18 months to 7 years:* use half the strength.
* *Children aged 7–14 years:* use half at age 7, increasing to the full dosage at age 14.
* *Newborn babies:* avoid using on very young or premature babies unless under the direction of a trained aromatherapist.

Note: On children it is wise to avoid the stronger essential oils unless specifically recommended. On babies it is advisable to stick to either lavender or chamomile essential oils.

MASSAGE TECHNIQUES
There are various types of movement used in massage:
* *Effleurage:* The basic stroking movements of massage which vary in pressure from the very light to really quite firm pressure. Generally the whole hand is used, but for different effects the heel of the hand or the

fingers can be used. A simple and natural technique, yet one which is very effective. Good as an initial treatment to warm and relax the muscles.

* *Petrissage:* A massage technique that uses kneading and wringing movements to reach deeper, working on muscles, ligaments and the connective tissue to release areas of tension. Works better on the fleshier areas of the body such as the hips, stomach and thighs. Use the hands alternatively to lift the tissues and knead them in a similar way to kneading bread.

* *Tapotement:* A tapping movement made by cupping the hands and gently slapping the body to produce a clapping sound. A quick, invigorating method of bringing fresh blood supplies to the surface of the skin. Very similar to Do-In, the traditional oriental form of self-massage, based on tapping the body from top to toe. Designed to get the circulation going, this is an excellent way to wake the body at the start the day.

* *Lymphatic Drainage:* This uses long sweeping movements, with the palms of the hands following the lymphatic channels in the body in a direction towards the lymph nodes. These are situated behind the knees, in the groin, under the arms, and beside the collarbones. The idea is to help drain away the toxins and impurities that collect in the lymphatic system. Lymphatic drainage is a useful technique for anyone with fluid retention, cellulite or skin disorders.

* *Reflexology:* Mainly used on the feet where there are several hundred 'reflex zones', but these are also found in the hands and ears. Reflex zones are nerve endings that correspond to areas and organs of the body. The theory is that by stimulating these zones you automatically stimulate the different parts of the body. Reflexology massage is easy to do: use the tips of the

thumbs to press lightly over the toes and sole of each foot, or the fingers and palms of each hand.

HOW TO GIVE A BODY MASSAGE

This is only a simplified guide and massages vary immensely depending on both the giver and receiver of the massage. It may sometimes be better, or more convenient, to massage only one area of the body. For instance when one area needs particular attention – the thighs and hips when treating cellulite, or the feet to pay particular attention to the reflex zones, or simply to give yourself a quick facial massage. If you do not feel like giving a complete body massage, a good area to concentrate on is the back. This is because the back and shoulders are where most people 'store' their tension. Massages are wonderful to give, but even better to receive. However, if there is no one around to oblige, do not forget that self-massage still has the benefits of aromatherapy. Children and babies love beneficial massages and it can establish a particularly special contact with them (remember to make up a more dilute oil blend, see page 49–50).

As touch is so powerful a communicator the mental state of the giver is extremely important. The mood of the giver sets the tone of the massage and thoughts should be of caring, nurturing and healing. It is good to try and work intuitively, 'listening' to the area of the body that is being worked upon. This means feeling the state of the muscles, noticing areas which are tense or knotted and then working on them until the tension eases. You should never rub so hard that it causes pain. Although sometimes massage can cause a type of ache, this should be the pleasant, healing ache of muscles letting go. Relax while giving a massage and try to work rhythmically with unhurried movements. It is important to have a warm room with a comfortable surface for the person to lie or sit upon. Also, arrange for a period of time free from any distractions, ideally followed by a quiet time to obtain the maximum effect.

To begin, pour some of the massage oil into the palm of your hand. A rough guide to the amount is to fill the hollow of the hand without overflowing, or enough to enable the hands to glide smoothly over the skin without slipping. Rub this between your hands to warm the oil before applying gently to the area which you will be working on.

The back of the person
Lie the person flat on their front with their arms by their side.

* **The Upper Back:** Position yourself at the head.
    1. Start with long, firm, stroking movements, using the palms or the heels of your hands. Let the hands travel down the back either side of the spine, outwards and up the side of the ribs, feeling for differences in tension and smoothing them out.
    2. Follow this by kneading the tissues of the neck and shoulders between finger and thumb, or with the whole hand; this must be done gently on this very sensitive area. Continue all around and across the shoulder blades.
    3. Using the thumbs, search for and apply pressure on any tense spots across the shoulders and down either side of the spine.
    4. Apply a series of strokes with the heels of both hands from the spine outwards on either side, working up and down the upper back.

* **The Lower Back:** Move to the side.
    1. Using kneading and wringing techniques work all over the lower back and waist area. Also include the buttocks.
    2. Pay special attention to the upper buttock region, as the muscles in this area can often be tense and may be sensitive. Work on this area with the heel of your hand and then searchingly with your thumbs.

3. Use whole-hand strokes down the area following the direction of the spine and then outwards across the back.

* **The Thigh:** Move level with the knees. Support the lower leg with a pillow or your own knee (if kneeling down) so that the person's knee is slightly bent.
   1. Knead and wring the tissues all round the thigh working from the knee up to the hip, paying particular attention to the outside of the upper leg.
   2. Use strong rhythmical strokes with both hands along the length from knee to buttock.

* **The Lower Leg:** Move down to the ankles and feet, again with the leg supported.
   1. Work as on the thighs, beginning with a kneading action, and then a rhythmic stroking up the leg.

* **The Foot:** Pick the foot up and support it with one hand while working on it with the other.
   1. Use your thumb to work over the sole of the foot with a slow, strong pressure, especially under the arch of the foot. The sole of the foot is where most of the reflex zones are, so working this area benefits the whole human body. Include the toes and the back of the ankle.

The front of the person

Lie the person flat on their back with both arms by their side.

* **The Foot:** Position yourself below the feet. Hold the foot with both hands, with the fingers under the sole and the thumb lying along the top.
   1. Gently pull your thumbs apart across the foot to stretch it, working up and down the foot.
   2. Work with your thumbs around the multitude of over-worked ankle bones and ligaments.

* **The Shin:** This area is very sensitive so it is important to work carefully, avoiding causing pain.
  1. Use a stroking technique both up the length and outwards across the muscles alongside the shinbone.
* **The Thigh:** Move up to the knees.
  1. Use your thumbs to work around the kneecap.
  2. Wring and knead the muscles from the centre to the side of the thigh.
  3. Stroke upwards from the knee to the hip.
  4. Using the whole hand work over, up and around the hip joint.
* **The Abdomen:** Move to one side of the waist.
  1. Circle both hands alternately around the abdominal area, going clockwise down the left-hand side of the body, just inside the left hip bone, across and up the right-hand side. Try to keep one hand always in contact with the body – as one hand leaves the body the other has already started its stroke. This movement follows the direction of the large intestine and is therefore particularly useful for easing indigestion and other digestive problems.
  2. Slide the hands down the rib cage using whole hand contact.
  3. Apply a very gentle pressure on the diaphragm with the whole hand below the breast bone.
* **The Chest:** Position yourself beside the head. Avoid the breasts unless requested when working on a female.
  1. Using the whole or the heel of the hand stretch the muscles outwards from the centre.
  2. Gently knead the area, including the muscles that run up into the shoulder from the breastbone. Remember to work gently on this sensitive area.
  3. Finish the chest with a series of long contact strokes, maybe slow circular movements.

* **The Arm:** Move to the side of the person and cradle and support the arm.
  1. Work the hand as you did the foot, using your thumbs and paying most attention to the palms.
  2. Knead and wring the tissues both along and across the arm.
  3. Use long, slow strokes along the length of the arm, from wrist to shoulder.
* **The Shoulder:** Remain beside the person.
  1. Use the heel or the whole of the hand to gently knead all over the shoulder.
  2. Place one hand on the front inside of the shoulder to hold it still, place the other hand on the outside of the shoulder with the fingers underneath and gently lift and circle the shoulder.
  3. From the head of the person place the hands under the shoulders, just either side of the neck, and massage with a circular movement.
  4. Place the hands under the back of the neck and gently vibrate them.
  5. Gently stretch the neck by putting upwards pressure on the base of the skull.
* **The Face:** Move to above the person's head.
  1. Begin with long sweeping strokes from the base of the neck, over the face and into the hairline.
  2. Use your fingertips to gently massage this entire area from the base of the neck up in small, circular movements. Pay particular attention to the jawline, cheeks and temples. If there is no objection to getting oil in the hair, include the scalp.
  3. Use your fingertips to massage the forehead from the centre outwards, with small, precise, pressing movements. Also press along the brow bones, just below the eyebrows.

4. Press along the jawline, working from the centre of the chin out to the ears.

5. Use the tips of your index fingers to firmly stroke outwards along the eyebrows, gently completing the circle around the eye socket.

6. Again using your index fingers, firmly stroke a curved line from the inner corner of your eye to your ear lobes, following the slope of the cheek-bones.

7. With light patting movements, gently tap the entire face and neck working upwards from the collar-bones.

* Finish the massage by returning to the feet and stroking them firmly along their length. Then place your hands flat on the soles of the feet for a few seconds. When the massage is over, leave your patient for a few minutes to allow him or her to come back to reality in their own time.

MASSAGE DURING PREGNANCY

It is a good idea to consult a trained aromatherapist and especial care must be taken with the choice of essential oils as many should be avoided during pregnancy (see page 62). A good mix of essential oils to use is tangerine combined with geranium. In the early stages of pregnancy when it is still possible to lie on the abdomen, the massage is the same as before, taking care to be very gentle when working on the abdominal area. For the more advanced stages of pregnancy, sit the mother-to-be on the edge of a bed to massage the neck and back, with a stool under the feet and a pillow on the lap on which to rest the arms. To massage the front of the body, have her lie down with pillows under the head and legs. The only action on the abdomen should be a gentle clockwise rubbing movement, or stroking.

Other Methods

BATH

Probably the easiest method of using essential oils. Run the bath – not too hot, because heat breaks down the structure of the oils and they cannot be absorbed if the skin is perspiring. Add either a single or mixture of oils, (generally not more than a combination of four) to the bath and stir the water well to disperse the drops. If using more than one oil they can be premixed or simply dropped into the bath water individually. Close the doors and windows so the vapours do not escape. Step in – relax and enjoy for ten minutes or more. To make a truly luxurious treat, combine your aromatic bath with candle light and some relaxing music.

Dosage

* *Adults:* Up to a maximum of eight drops.
* *Children:* Up to a maximum of four drops.
* *Babies (below 18 months):* One to two drops. (*Note:* This is the dosage for a full-sized bath, not a baby bath.)

SHOWER

Wash as usual. Add the essential oil to a sponge or flannel and rub over the entire body while standing under the running water. Breathe deeply to inhale the vapours.

Dosage

* *Adults:* A maximum of eight drops, but four to five drops should be sufficient.
* Not recommended for children.

FOOTBATH

Add the essential oils to a bowl of hot water (not scorching) and soak the feet for ten minutes. A variation on a simple footbath is to put around fifteen to twenty smooth pebbles or marbles in the bottom of the bowl. Then, as the feet are soaking, gently move them back and forth across the pebbles. This massages the feet effectively and also stimulates the many reflex zones.

Dosage

* Maximum of five drops in a washing-up-sized bowl.

INHALATION

One method is to add the essential oils to a bowl of steaming water (just off the boil). Drape a towel over your head and the bowl to enclose the vapours. Close your eyes and inhale deeply through your nose for one to three minutes.

Dosage and safety

* Two to three drops in a large serving bowl.
* Discontinue if there is any discomfort.
* Exercise caution if you suffer from asthma or hay fever.

Alternatively, one to two drops of an essential oil on a handkerchief or tissue can be sniffed when required. Do not use essential oils directly on clothes as they may stain wool and other delicate fabrics. Tissue inhalations can be especially useful when travelling or as an instant tonic in stressful situations. A couple of drops of a calming oil, such as chamomile, can be dabbed onto the pillow at night to help induce sleep or relaxation.

DIFFUSERS AND VAPORISERS

These are a great alternative to artificial air fresheners. Essential oils go one better by being not simply nice smells, but also having all the therapeutic and cleansing benefits of aromatherapy. Diffusers and vaporisers are readily available in health and some gift shops. They vary in design from pretty night lights and electrical devices, to a simple metal or ceramic ring which sits on a light bulb. Be careful whenever using a burner with a naked flame as essential oils are highly flammable. Most work by heating a small amount of water and a couple of drops of essential oil. However, heat does change the structure of essential oils so although these fragrance the air, the therapeutic benefits are lost. The most effective type release the essential oils without heating them. Some diffusers achieve this with a small electric air pump to waft the pure essential oils into the atmosphere. These not only scent the room, but are also absorbed by the skin.

Home-made alternatives are easy and inexpensive to use. Simply place a small bowl of warm water with a couple of drops of your chosen essential oil in it near a radiator or other warm place. Alternatively tuck a tissue or cotton-wool ball which has been dampened with water and a few drops of essential oil behind the radiator. For a more immediate effect, take a plant-sprayer with some warm water and a couple of drops of essential oil and spray around the room – however be careful in rooms with wood furniture as the oils could mark surfaces.

NEAT

Essential oils should very rarely be used neat on the skin – never use them in this way unless it is specifically recommended. Lavender oil has an amazing healing effect on burns and reduces subsequent scarring, so it is a good oil to keep handy in the kitchen. Lavender or tea tree oil dabbed onto minor cuts or insect bites will soothe and act as an antiseptic. Apart from these minor uses in small amounts the application of neat essential oil should only be carried out by a qualified aromatherapist.

Dosage and safety

* Do not exceed the maximum neat dosage of two drops.
* Do not use an oil which is not recommended specifically for use neat.

INTERNAL USE

Some doctors, mainly in France, prescribe essential oils to be taken orally with water; but essential oils should never be taken by mouth unless under the supervision of a highly qualified practitioner. Like any other concentrated extract, they can damage the mucous membranes of the mouth, cause stomach damage and even liver poisoning. However, even when prescribed, taking the oils internally is actually less effective than absorbing them through the skin, and we miss out on all the benefits to be had from smelling them. Essential oils are also used in very small amounts as flavourings in food and drink, for example bergamot in Earl Grey tea, peppermint in mint creams and lemon in both sweet and savory dishes.

Safety

* Never take internally unless prescribed by a qualified practitioner.

Health Warnings:

* Never take essential oils by mouth unless under medical instructions.
  IF AN ESSENTIAL OIL IS ACCIDENTALLY SWALLOWED: Drink as much water as possible and seek immediate medical attention.
* Keep essential oils away from the eyes.
  IF AN ESSENTIAL OIL IS ACCIDENTALLY SPLASHED IN THE EYES: This will cause pain and irritation. Flush with plenty of water, several times. If the pain does not subside, consult your doctor.
* Do not apply neat essential oils to the skin, unless specifically indicated.
  IF A NEAT ESSENTIAL OIL IS ACCIDENTALLY SPLASHED ONTO THE SKIN: Wash well with plenty of water. If there is continued irritation seek medical attention.
* People who suffer from allergies or sensitive skin should always patch-test each essential oil or blend before using widely.

IF THE SKIN IS IRRITATED: wash well with plenty of water; if it continues seek medical attention.

* People suffering from advanced asthmatic conditions, epilepsy, heart conditions, varicose veins, or any acute illness or condition should seek medical advice before using essential oils.

* People taking homeopathic remedies should check with their practitioner before using essential oils. This is because the strong aromas may cancel the effects of some homeopathic remedies.

* Essential oils should be used with great care during pregnancy as they enter the bloodstream and may cross the placental barrier. Aromatherapy is however a wonderful treatment for the mum-to-be and very useful during pregnancy and labour. It is advisable to consult a qualified aromatherapist.

Essential oils to be avoided during pregnancy:

Basil
Clary sage
Hyssop
Juniper berry
Marjoram
Myrrh
Pine
Rosemary
Sage
Thyme

Essential oils that have been recommended by aromatherapists for use during pregnancy:

Chamomile
Citrus oils, eg. tangerine and grapefruit
Geranium
Lavender
Neroli
Rose
Sandalwood

Remember that toxicity is purely a matter of dosage. Many substances we eat or apply to our bodies would in extremely large quantities be toxic. The dosages and cautions given here err on the side of overcaution. This is important for safety's sake, but do not let the guidelines deter you from the many benefits to be gained by using essential oils for health and well-being.

—6—
Recipe Blending

Here are a few simple essential oil recipe blends for many different purposes. There is, however, no reason why you cannot adapt these to suit your own individual needs or taste, or even make up your own recipes.

Blissful Bath Oils

THE GREAT UNWINDER
Relax after a really hard day and ease tense, aching shoulder muscles:
  4 drops cypress
  2 drops lavender
  2 drops cajuput

QUICK PICK-ME-UP
Let those blues just float away.
  4 drops lemon
  4 drops ylang ylang

THE ENERGISER
Need an extra bit of help to get up and go?
  4 drops tangerine
  4 drops bergamot

THE APHRODISIAC
Ideal for a night of passion – or simply to make you feel special.
  4 drops patchouli
  2 drops ylang ylang
  2 drops jasmine

IMMUNE SYSTEM STRENGTHENER
To prevent feeling under the weather as the winter months set in, or whenever your defences are low.
  4 drops tea tree
  2 drops lavender
  2 drops eucalyptus

THE COMFORTER

Make a hot drink, put on
your favourite music and
wallow in the aroma.

4 drops sandalwood
2 drops bergamot
2 drops clary sage

Marvellous Massage Oils

BASIC BODY OIL

An excellent every day oil that
will moisturise the skin after
bathing.

50ml grapeseed oil
5ml wheatgerm oil
10 drops lavender
10 drops chamomile

THE ULTIMATE RELAXING BLEND

A wonderful blend for combating the effects of stress and
restoring a sense of well-
being. Concentrate on massaging the knots out of the shoulders, which is where most of
us tend to hold our tension.

50ml grapeseed oil.
5ml wheatgerm oil
8 drops neroli
8 drops sandalwood
4 drops rosemary

REFRESHMENT

This massage will refresh the
senses and uplift the mood. A
lovely way to start the
weekend after a hard week's
work.

50ml grapeseed oil
5ml wheatgerm oil
10 drops tangerine
5 drops lemon
5 drops geranium

STIMULATING FORMULATION

A refreshing body oil that will
wake up the senses in the
morning and which has a
non-sticky texture, so can be
used before getting dressed.
Great for use before exercise
to warm up the muscles.

50ml grapeseed oil
5ml wheatgerm oil
10 drops cajuput
10 drops peppermint

AFTER-SPORT MUSCLE RUB

This invigorating lotion is excellent for reviving a flagging physique and smells macho enough for the fussiest male! Apply liberally to the muscles which have been working the hardest.

50ml grapeseed oil
5ml wheatgerm oil
8 drops rosemary
8 drops cedarwood
4 drops eucalyptus

REMOISTURISING BODY OIL

This soothing oil can be used for massage and a splash may also be added to the bath if the skin is very dry. Especially good for areas of hardened, chapped skin on the hands, elbows and feet, as the avocado oil penetrates the surface layer of skin to moisturise below.

25ml avocado oil
25ml almond oil
5ml wheatgerm oil
10 drops chamomile
5 drops sandalwood
5 drops frankincense

For a lighter, yet nourishing oil for dry skin, substitute grape-seed oil for the avocado. This version would be useful as a general massage oil on sensitive skin and could also be used to treat eczema.

PAMPERING PREGNANCY

A nourishing blend useful for helping prevent stretch marks and inducing a general feeling of well-being and relaxation in pregnancy. Lightly stroke the abdomen and avoid vigorous massage.

50ml almond oil
5ml wheatgerm oil
4 drops lavender
4 drops sandalwood
2 drops tangerine
2 drops geranium

ANTI-CELLULITE OIL

This formula is highly effective at helping to break down the fatty deposits that lead to the dimpled, orange-peel effect on hips and thighs. Use daily on the hips and buttocks after bathing, massaging into the skin with firm, circular movements.

50ml grapeseed oil
5ml wheatgerm oil
10 drops juniper
10 drops lemon
5 drops cypress

THE FEMININE OIL

Suffer from PMT or irregular periods? Try this general massage blend for minor gynaecological problems. Use daily on the abdomen and lower back.

25ml grapeseed oil
25ml almond oil
5ml wheatgerm oil
8 drops chamomile
8 drops marjoram
4 drops neroli

SPOTTY BACK MASSAGE OIL

An excellent, lightweight oil for clearing up spots and pimples on the back and shoulders.

50ml jojoba oil
10 drops tea tree
10 drops lavender

AFTER-SUN SOOTHING OIL

A suntan is simply a sign of damaged skin and the sun is one of the main factors in skin ageing. However, you can repair some of the damage caused by the sun's rays with this nourishing oil, as it has a high vitamin E content which will help minimise free radical cell damage.

25ml grapeseed oil
25ml extra virgin olive oil
15ml wheatgerm oil
10 drops chamomile
5 drops bergamot
5 drops myrrh

WINTER BUG ZAPPER

A wonderfully invigorating and cleansing blend to help stave off those miserable winter chills, coughs and colds.

25ml jojoba oil
25ml grapeseed oil
5ml wheatgerm oil
8 drops pine
8 drops eucalyptus
4 drops tea tree

Fabulous Facial Oils

FOR NORMAL SKIN
This blend is an excellent all-round face massage oil. Add a couple of drops of tangerine in the morning.

> 25ml jojoba oil
> 25ml peach-nut or apricot-kernel oil
> 5ml wheatgerm oil
> 10 drops lavender
> 5 drops geranium
> 5 drops neroli

FOR DRY SKIN
> 25ml avocado oil
> 25ml peach-nut/apricot-kernel oil
> 10ml wheatgerm oil
> 10 drops sandalwood
> 5 drops geranium
> 5 drops rose

FOR COMBINATION SKIN
> 50ml jojoba oil
> 10 drops lavender
> 10 drops cedarwood

FOR OILY SKIN
> 50ml jojoba oil
> 10 drops patchouli
> 5 drops lemon
> 5 drops cypress

FOR MATURE SKIN
This richer blend makes an excellent night-time treatment.

> 25ml almond oil
> 25ml jojoba oil
> 5ml wheatgerm oil
> 10ml evening primrose oil (or the contents of 4 capsules)
> 10 drops frankincense
> 10 drops geranium

FOR DEVITALISED SKIN
A good tonic for tired and stressed skins.

> 25ml jojoba oil
> 25ml peach-nut/apricot-kernel oil
> 10ml wheat-germ oil
> 5 drops lavender
> 5 drops neroli
> 5 drops jasmine

TO HELP ACNE
Put those pimples in a panic with this effective anti-acne blend.

> 50ml jojoba oil
> 10 drops cypress
> 5 drops tea tree
> 5 drops patchouli

PEPPERMINT
SKIN SOLUTION

A useful treatment for spotty and acne-prone skins. Dab this easy-to-make oil on the affected area twice daily.

> 10ml hazelnut or jojoba oil
> 1 drop peppermint
> 1 drop tea tree

REFRESHING SPRITZER

This instant skin refresher is especially useful during hot weather. Place all the ingredients in a screw-top bottle or jar and shake well. Transfer the liquid to a plastic spray bottle with a fine mist pump (available from chemists and good department stores). Store in the fridge and use to lightly spritz over the face and neck. Can be sprayed over foundation and powder to set it in place.

> 100ml fizzy (carbonated) mineral water
> 2 drops peppermint
> 3 drops neroli

FLORAL WATER

This is a deliciously perfumed tonic water which is ideal to splash onto the face after cleansing or to spray over make-up to set it in place. Remember to shake it before each use.

> 100ml still mineral water
> 5 drops lavender
> 5 drops neroli

Handy Help

Hand massage helps keep the hands soft, supple and smooth, and this blend is light enough to use every day. Sesame and almond oil contain mild natural sunscreens and will act as a filter against the damaging effects of the sun that can cause liver spots. The essential oils are added mainly for fragrance but will also soothe dryer, more mature skins. For a more intensive treatment, massage a generous amount into the hands and cuticles, slip on a pair of cotton gloves and leave overnight. By the morning your hands will feel like new (cotton gloves are available at good glove counters).

50ml jojoba oil
50ml sesame or almond oil
10 drops sandalwood
10 drops rose

Seasonal Scents

These four great mixtures are for room diffusers or burners. Give your home or office an instant lift. All of these recipes give a total of ten drops, so remember to vary the amount depending on the method of diffusion or vaporisation used.

SIMPLY SPRING

6 drops lemon
2 drops lavender
2 drops bergamot

SUMMER SUNSHINE

4 drops geranium
4 drops petitgrain
2 drops rose

AUTUMNAL WARMTH

5 drops sandalwood
3 drops cajuput
2 drops rosemary

WINTER WELCOME

4 drops frankincense
4 drops mandarin
2 drops pine

Aromatherapy Home Help

From looking after your own health, to gardening, caring for pets, cleaning the house, or simply making life smell good – essential oils have a million and more uses. Many such areas of usage are quite deserving of a book in their own right. Here I thought it might be interesting to touch on a few simple ideas. But you can easily experiment – the only limit is your imagination.

Ideal Presents

Stuck for something to give? Run out of novel and individual ideas? Look no further. A lovely idea is to give an aromatherapy 'starter kit' – all that's needed is a few of the essential oils (see the recommended basic kit list on page 23). Add one or two carrier oils, pack them into a little basket or box, maybe with some shredded tissue paper and ribbons. Alternatively, buy a diffuser or vaporiser and pop in a couple of your favourite essential oils. An economical as well as thoughtful and personal gift is to make up a bath or massage blend – perhaps one of your own tried and tested mixtures, or one designed especially with someone in mind. Some real fun is to be had when thinking up names for your inventions. For those who enjoy sewing, essential oils can add another dimension to your creations – sprinkle a few drops on the stuffing of a cushion to create an aromatic pillow or in the stuffing of a soft toy (the soothing essence of lavender oil in a favourite teddy-bear could make parents very grateful!).

If the creative streak in you takes hold, it can be applied to many kinds of different areas. A couple of drops of a carefully chosen essential oil will give the final product just a touch of extra and invisible appeal (remember to take care when working with delicate fabrics or good wood as they might become marked). For a quick and completely hassle-free present, give someone a treatment with a professional aromatherapist. Many aromatherapists offer their own gift vouchers, or would certainly allow for a session to be paid for in advance. An aromatherapy session suits everyone, although you may have to answer for getting someone hooked on the wondrous world of aromatherapy! Some aromatherapists can even arrange home visits – especially useful for the elderly and new mums.

Post the Aroma

Perfumed paper takes on a new dimension when you consider posting a whiff of aromatherapy. Chamomile for a depressed friend, geranium or sandalwood for a stressed colleague and marjoram for someone who has suffered a setback. Not all letters are to those with problems, but how nice it would be to give someone a refreshing burst of tangerine as they open their morning post on the way to work. And yes, with those love letters you could always go over the top and add the aphrodisiacal ylang ylang. Simply dab the corner of the paper with a touch of your chosen essential oil before sealing your mobile aromatherapy in its envelope. Gift vouchers for aromatherapy sessions are also easy to post and are always well received.

Let's Party

Putting the guests into the right frame of mind is the secret of any good party, so why not use all the methods at your disposal? Create the right atmosphere for your party whatever your style – from a frenetic bop, through a lazy afternoon, to a romantic dinner for two. Geranium and melissa with a hint of lemon should both relax and invigorate, helping the conversation along in those tricky beginning moments. For a headier relaxing atmosphere combine clary sage with exotic ylang ylang. For a dinner party, light the candles beforehand and once the wax around the wick has melted, place a drop of an essential oil in each one (be careful though – remember that all essential oils are flammable). You could pick an oil that would complement or balance the food. For that heavy gastronomic feast, create a light, tangy atmosphere with tangerine, or the warmth of rosewood or cypress to accompany a mediterranean-style menu.

For seasonal celebrations, a couple of well-chosen aromas will get anyone in the mood. The majority of us will have some 'fragrance memories' of Christmas and the right aroma will soften up the most determined Scrooge. Tangerine, pine, cedarwood and frankincense are all evocative of the traditional family Christmas. At this time of year, make use of a real fire. Take a couple of pieces of the wood or coal and put a drop of essential oil on each one and leave to soak for half an hour. Light the fire, sit back and let the aromatic aroma waft over your Christmas frivolities. Going to someone else's party? Remember that essential oils are ideal to get you in the party mood before you arrive!

Post-Party Blues

Unfortunately, there is no complete cure for a hangover except abstinence the night before. However, there is a case for damage limitation. Nothing is as effective as drinking several large glasses of water but, in addition, a mixture of juniper with lavender and a hint of sandalwood would make an excellent relaxing bath or massage. The diuretic properties of this blend will help the body to flush the effects of the alcohol out of your system. For those who have to get up early and continue with a hectic schedule, try a combination of reviving rosemary and tangerine in your morning bath or shower. If the problem has also been caused by an over-indulgence in all those rich heavy foods try massaging the abdomen with a blend with juniper, lemon and a hint of marjoram. Use firm gentle strokes in a clockwise direction (see page 54). This will encourage your digestive system to operate far more effectively and disperse trapped wind or heartburn.

Home Sweet Home

It does not need a special occasion to motivate us into making our homes more welcoming places. It is something we can all do for our nearest and dearest, or as an indulgent treat for ourselves. Warm and comforting smells for the hall in winter, refreshing scents for the summer, a relaxing fragrance in the bedroom and invigorating aromas in the kitchen. Pick the fragrances you particularly love to make your home that little bit special. Trying to sell your property? Some unobtrusive aromatherapy never did anyone any harm. Before you have viewers around, use a vaporiser or diffuser to create an attractive ambience. Use lemon for a clean, refreshing smell that will help revive the most jaded house buyer, or try sandalwood for a comforting, homely aroma that will calm and relax. Try different aromas in different rooms, but remember subtlety is the key. Our nose is a sensitive organ, though, so don't overdo it.

Household Hints

Loathe the washing-up? Buy unperfumed washing-up liquid and add ten drops of an essential oil. Otherwise add a couple of drops to the washing-up water so you can bury your hands in aromatic suds to suit the mood of the moment. The citrus oils are to be particularly recommended, but patchouli could add a touch of the exotic and peppermint is especially refreshing.

How about cleaning? Lovely smells, very hygienic (remember the antiseptic properties of the essential oils) and kind to your skin. Add a couple of drops of an essential oil to the final rinse water, or a drop directly on a damp cloth when cleaning a whole range of surfaces. Ideal in the kitchen and bathroom, or even when cleaning the paintwork and the windows.

Essential oils can even be used when washing clothes. By hand, add a drop to the final rinse water. In the machine simply place three drops in with the fabric softener. In the tumble dryer, alternatively, pop in a scrap of material with a couple of drops sprinkled on it. So have your T-shirts smelling of refreshing tangerine, the kid's nightshirts of relaxing lavender, men's shirts of macho sandalwood and your underwear of rose otto.

Scented Insect Repellents

After having for years suffered the nasty niffs of chemical insect repellents, it comes as a surprise to find that the horrible beasties can be effectively kept away by far more pleasant means. This method also does not pollute our homes and atmosphere with toxic chemicals. Use a vaporiser or diffuser. If eating outside on warm sunny nights, use an aromatic candle as a beautiful centrepiece (carefully add a couple of drops of oil to the wax round the wick once it has begun to melt). If the insect's passage of entry is a regularly used trail, a couple of drops of essential oil on the route works wonders. For windows, some drops sprinkled onto strips of cotton ribbon or paper towelling hung down from the top does the trick.

Essential oils to use as good all-round deterrents are: lavender (especially for flies and moths), peppermint and lemon (good for mosquitoes and ants), basil, rosewood and thyme. Moths also have an aversion to citrus oils. A marvellous alternative to your winter coats and woollens smelling of mothballs is to use scraps of material impregnated with a mixture of a citrus oil and lavender.

Remedy Finder

Aches and Pains

General – massage the affected area.

basil, bay, cedarwood, clary sage, eucalyptus, hyssop, juniper, marjoram, pine, rosemary, tangerine

Arthritis – attacks at the joints with inflammation, pain, stiffness, loss of mobility and, eventually, permanent damage to joint surfaces. A principal cause is excess uric acid deposited in the joint spaces. Aromatherapy massage operates by trying to break down these deposits. The joints usually affected are either those which have been subjected to a lot of stress through sport, dance, physical work or obesity, or those which are the site of an earlier injury.

bergamot, hyssop, lavender, marjoram, peppermint, rosemary

Cramp – an involuntary and painful contraction of a single muscle or group of muscles. Cramps can be caused by chilling, or from loss of body salts after vomiting, sweating or diarrhoea. However they often occur for no apparent reason. Massage of the affected area brings rapid relief.

clary sage, cypress, juniper, marjoram, rosemary

Headaches – literally an ache in the head. Caused by a wide variety of factors from fatigue to continuous noise –

chamomile, eucalyptus, lavender,

virtually everyone will suffer from a *peppermint,*
headache at some point. Using essential *rosemary*
oils to relieve a headache is far kinder
on the body than reaching for the
bottle of aspirin. A mixture of lavender
and peppermint in equal proportions is
very effective. For a quick remedy, rub
a drop of neat lavender onto the
temples.

Migraine – a severe one-sided headache, *basil, chamomile,*
generally accompanied by one or more *eucalyptus, lavender,*
of the following symptoms: nausea; *peppermint*
dizziness; extreme sensitivity to light,
touch, noise or smell; loss of vision.
Aromatherapy is better used as a
preventative measure due to acute sensitivity during an attack. Often caused by
stress or trigger foods.

Rheumatism – inflammation of the muscles *bay, cypress,*
and joints, with acute pain and *eucalyptus, hyssop,*
swelling. The essential oils operate by *juniper, lavender,*
bringing some relief from the pain and *marjoram, pine,*
helping to eliminate the build up of *rosemary, sage, thyme*
uric acid and other toxins which are
often involved in rheumatic conditions.

Sprains – a joint injury in which the liga- *bay, chamomile,*
ment has been damaged. The joint will *lavender, marjoram,*
be swollen, painful, and possibly hot to *rosemary, sage*
touch. The injury should not be
massaged but essential oils can be
added to water while bathing the joint,
or applied in a cold compress.
Follow this with a supporting bandage
and rest.

Strained muscles – this is an injury due to misuse or overuse of muscles, generally through sport, dance or physical work. The best cure for strained muscles is rest, but aromatherapy can be useful – especially oils added to a warm bath, to aid relaxation.

juniper, marjoram, melissa, thyme

Circulatory Problems

Chilblains – found mainly in the feet, but also in the hands. These are characterised by swelling, itching and redness. They are caused by a combination of poor blood circulation and extreme coldness constricting and reducing the supply of oxygen to the skin. Marjoram and juniper work well as an immediate treatment to improve the circulation.

chamomile, cypress, juniper, lavender, lemon, marjoram, rosemary

High blood pressure – as a continued state, high blood pressure places strain on the heart, blood vessels and the kidneys. It generally affects those people who are extremely stressed and find it hard to relax. Massage with calming, soothing and relaxing oils can be a most effective way of lowering the blood pressure. However this is a serious condition and the entire life style should be examined and changes made.

clary sage, hyssop, lavender, lemon, marjoram, rosemary, thyme, ylang ylang

Poor circulation – may lead to poor skin tone, feeling cold and tiring easily, and even to fainting. A vigorous massage boosts the most sluggish circulation and encourages blood flow.

cypress, geranium, hyssop, juniper, lemon, mandarin, marjoram, neroli, pine, rose, rosemary, thyme

Colds, 'Flu, Respiratory Disorders, etc.

Asthma – attacks of tight-chested wheeziness and difficulty with breathing. Physically they are muscle spasms in the narrow passages of the lungs. Due to the reduced air flow, there is often a build up of mucus making the condition even worse. Attacks can be triggered by allergies, pollutants, cold air, infections such as the common cold, and stress or acute anxiety.

Aromatherapy is more useful as an ongoing preventative measure. Massage the shoulders, back and chest with the intention of relaxing the muscles and promoting deep breathing.

cedarwood, clary sage, eucalyptus, hyssop, lavender, marjoram

Bronchitis – the symptoms are an aching throat, tight chest, cough, headache, and probably a temperature. It is caused by an inflammation of the bronchial tubes. In the earlier stages, when the cough is drier, steam inhalations are particularly useful. In the later stages when the mucus is beginning to move more freely, the oils should be applied via baths and specific massages to the chest and throat.

basil, cedarwood, eucalyptus, frankincense, marjoram, myrrh, sage, tangerine, tea tree

Catarrh – the production of excessive mucus in the nose and respiratory passages. Results from inflammation of the mucus membrane that lines these passages, which can be caused by infections or irritants such as pollen and

bergamot, cedarwood, eucalyptus, lemon, pine, rosemary, sage, sandalwood

house dust. In some, sensitivity to a particular food (often dairy products) can be the problem. For immediate relief, use a steam inhalation. To help drain mucus from the sinuses, use gentle but firm facial massage.

Colds – the common cold is just that – common! Regular aromatherapy offers relief by warding off the bugs with anti-septic oils and helps prevent potentially worse secondary infections. Use essential oils in baths and steam inhalations.   *basil, bay, cajuput, cypress, eucalyptus, frankincense, hyssop, lavender, marjoram, pine, tea tree*

Coughs – these are the body's natural action to rid the mucous membrane of the throat and upper respiratory tract of an irritation such as dust, smoke or excessive mucus. They should not therefore be suppressed. The most appropriate aromatherapy treatment is a steam inhalation. Localised massage to the throat and chest and room diffusers are also useful.   *bergamot, cedarwood, cypress, eucalyptus, frankincense, hyssop, juniper, lavender, lemon, marjoram, sandalwood*

'Flu – more properly influenza, is the term given to a number of similar virus infections, some of them still unidenti-fied. The symptoms are that of a severe cold, together with a temperature and aching limbs. Take a warm bath at the first sign of 'flu, adding tea tree essen-tial oil, and go straight to bed. Regular use of essential oils in the bath can strengthen the immune system and make us less susceptible to the many 'flu viruses.   *bay, eucalyptus, lavender, tea tree*

Laryngitis – acute inflammation of the larynx, resulting in hoarseness or complete loss of voice. Caused by infection or irritation (including excessive shouting). Steam inhalations offer rapid relief.

frankincense, jasmine, lavender, sandalwood, thyme

Respiratory disorders – massage the chest, back and shoulders with the intention of relaxing the muscles and encouraging deep breathing. Steam inhalations also help bring relief.

bay, cedarwood, eucalyptus, hyssop, myrrh, pine, sandalwood, thyme

Sinusitis – inflammation of the sinuses, leading to congestion. The sinuses are the cavities above, behind and to the sides of the nose. Sinusitis can give rise to severe earache and headache. Frequent steam inhalations are effective at easing this problem.

eucalyptus, peppermint, pine, tea tree, thyme

Sore throat – discomfort which can be caused by a virus or bacterial infection. Often eased with a series of steam inhalations. A very effective remedy is to gargle with a single drop of thyme essential oil in half a tumbler of water, remembering to spit it out afterwards. Localised massage with diluted thyme essential oil is also very soothing and fights the infection.

clary sage, eucalyptus, geranium, hyssop, lavender, lemon, pine, thyme

Digestive and Urinary Problems

basil, bergamot, juniper, lemon, mandarin, marjoram, melissa, myrrh, peppermint, sage, tangerine

Digestive – for general discomfort, massage the upper abdomen in a clockwise direction.

∗ *Constipation* – the most common causes of which are poor diet, stress, or lack of exercise. Massage the lower abdomen, always in a clockwise direction.

marjoram, rosemary, tangerine, ylang ylang

∗ *Diarrhoea* – repeated loose, soft or liquid stools, which may be caused by excitement, spicy or unusual foods, overeating or infection. Massage the lower abdomen gently and drink plenty of water to prevent dehydration.

chamomile, geranium, lavender, neroli, peppermint, rosemary

Urinary – for general complaints, use baths or massage with essential oils. But as with any problems with the urinary system, remember to drink plenty of water.

cypress, juniper, lavender

∗ *Cystitis* – inflammation of the urinary bladder, caused by bacteria. Urination is painful, often there is a burning sensation and, occasionally, discoloration of the urine with blood. Use essential oils in the bath and in a very dilute solution to wash the local area. Massage of the lower abdomen may also be helpful.

bergamot, cajuput, cypress, eucalyptus, juniper, lavender, sandalwood, tea tree, thyme

∗ *Bed wetting* – involuntary passing of urine at night. Use the essential oils in a quick massage or an aromatic bath before bed. Remember to reduce the dosages of essential oils for children in massage blends.

chamomile, cypress, lavender

∗ *Fluid retention* – can cause pain and discomfort. Best alleviated by

bergamot, cypress, juniper, mandarin,

regular massage, concentrating on the lymphatic drainage sites in the armpits, groin and behind the knees. *patchouli, pine, rosemary, sandalwood*

Travel sickness – nausea and possibly vomiting in response to the motion of a moving motor vehicle, boat or aeroplane. Take a tissue sprinkled with a couple of drops of lavender and peppermint essential oils and sniff as required. It may help to take a relaxing bath before leaving home. *ginger, lavender, lemon, peppermint*

Hormonal

Menstrual disorders – period pain is the most common problem. To relieve, gently massage the abdomen and, if possible, the lower back. The best essential oils for this are marjoram, lavender and chamomile. Another common problem is that of abnormally heavy periods, in which case geranium or rose essential oils can be of particular help. In fact, rose would be a great help to women who suffer from almost any period problems as it has a general regulating effect and is reputed to be a uterine tonic. For those who suffer from pre-menstrual tension (PMT), any of the antidepressant oils will help relieve general depression and irritability. The physical symptoms, which may include any combination of fluid *basil, cajuput, chamomile, clary sage, geranium, jasmine, juniper, marjoram, neroli, rose, sage, sandalwood, thyme*

retention, breast tenderness, swollen abdomen, headache and nausea can be treated with a gentle massage or a warm, relaxing bath. A combination of geranium and rosemary has been found to be effective at removing the worst of these symptoms.

Menopause – when women stop menstruating in their forties or fifties they may experience depression, hot flushes, irregular or excessively heavy periods and insomnia. Again, all the antidepressant oils may be pressed into service, with rose being particularly helpful.

clary sage, cypress, geranium, marjoram, neroli, rose

Post-natal depression – the depression which some women suffer after their babies are born is particularly sad at a time which one would like to remember as happy. The antidepressant oils can all be used in the bath. Being given a gentle massage at such a time can also be very helpful.

clary sage, lemon, melissa, neroli

Infections – General

Bacterial infections – all high quality essential oils will help inhibit the growth of a bacterial infection.

lavender, melissa, myrrh, sage, sandalwood, tea tree, thyme

Fever – a fever is basically a high temperature often accompanied by profuse sweating. It is an important, natural healing process of the body as it rids

bergamot, eucalyptus, frankincense, lemon, patchouli, peppermint

itself of toxins via perspiration. A couple of drops of essential oil in a bowl of cool water can be used to sponge the body to help reduce the temperature. However if the fever is not too bad, it is good to let the patient 'sweat it out'. A bath with tea tree essential oil followed by bed rest will be of immense help. When there is a high fever, massage should not be used.

Fungal infections – all the antifungal essential oils will be of help.

melissa, myrrh, patchouli, sandalwood, tea tree

* *Athlete's foot* – moist, itchy and often cracked skin between and around the toes. It may be useful to use the essential oils in an alcohol carrier (you may be able to buy an appropriate alcohol from the chemist, if not a small amount of vodka works well) until the skin has dried out, before switching to the more usual carrier oils.

lavender, lemon, myrrh, tea tree

* *Candidiasis* – infection of the mucous membrane by the fungus *Candida albicans*. The most common form is thrush, which is found in the vagina and lower intestinal tract. The fungus is actually present all the time in the gut, but the beneficial intestinal bacteria usually prevents it from proliferating to a problematic level. Baths are a particularly useful form of treatment.

lavender, myrrh, tea tree

Immune system – the human body is amazing – far more sophisticated than anything yet invented by mankind. The immune system is our early warning system to protect the body from illness and infection. These essential oils help strengthen this response – a useful course of action when there is no specific problem, or as a preventative measure during the winter months.

bergamot, cajuput, lavender, lemon, pine, rosemary, sandalwood, tea tree, thyme

Viral infections – a viral infection should be tackled at the first opportunity. A hot bath with tea tree essential oil can be particularly helpful.

bergamot, eucalyptus, hyssop, tea tree, thyme

Inflammation and Allergies

Allergies – for general use the essential oils which are calming and soothing are the best to treat allergic reactions. This can be of dual help as allergies can frequently be linked to stress. (See also asthma and eczema.)

chamomile, geranium, lavender, melissa

Hay fever – this is an allergic response to various pollens and so affects people most in mid-to-late summer. Symptoms include streaming eyes, runny nose and frequent sneezing.

chamomile, eucalyptus, juniper

Inflammation – in general this can be provoked by bacteria, injury or irritants and can give rise to pain, swelling and itching.

chamomile, eucalyptus, lavender, myrrh, peppermint, tea tree

Inflamed skin – see skin.

Insect bites/stings – where it is appropriate, make sure the sting is removed and then wash with a water dilution of the given oils. A couple of drops of lavender or tea tree can be dabbed on neat, to soothe and promote healing.

chamomile, lavender, lemon, tea tree

Mental Aids

Concentration – occasionally, we can all do with any help we can get to improve our concentration. Using room diffusers while working can be particularly useful.

basil, bergamot, cedarwood, frankincense, peppermint

Fatigue – essential oils can help lift fatigue for a while, but do not expect miracles. The only permanent cure is sleep! However, these oils are the most stimulating.

basil, clary sage, frankincense, lavender, rose, rosemary, thyme

Insomnia – difficulty with falling asleep. A relaxing bath before bed and a couple of drops of lavender essential oil on the pillow work wonders.

bay, chamomile, lavender, mandarin, marjoram, petitgrain

Lethargy – can be draining and self-perpetuating. Break the vicious circle with an uplifting massage blend.

jasmine, rosemary, tangerine, thyme

Sedative or tranquilliser – calming and composing, can be useful in cases of overexcitement and pain.

chamomile, clary sage, mandarin, melissa, sandalwood, ylang ylang

Tonic – the all-round general pick-me-up, for all ages and occasions.

lavender, lemon, mandarin, melissa, neroli, rosemary, tangerine, ylang ylang

Nervous System

Anxiety – a state of apprehension. A relaxing massage with calming essential oils can be particularly useful.

jasmine, lemon, mandarin, marjoram, myrrh, neroli, petitgrain, thyme, ylang ylang

Depression – aromatherapy is an excellent therapy to help relieve depression. When choosing essential oils, use the preferences of the particular person at that time as a guide. Aromatherapy in the bath is particularly useful as it is also a positive self-help method of medication.

bay, bergamot, clary sage, geranium, jasmine, neroli, petitgrain, rose, sage, sandalwood, tangerine, ylang ylang

Fainting – caused by a decreased blood supply to the brain. When we receive a great emotional shock or fright, the nervous system diverts a large amount of blood to the abdominal area, which can cause fainting. A 'faint' is normally very temporary, if a person loses consciousness for any length of time seek urgent medical attention.

lavender, neroli, peppermint

Hysteria – an outbreak of extreme wild emotion. Inhaling a calming essential oil can be useful. If the person is completely out of control, the easiest way may be to spray it around them. Once the initial hysteria has subsided, a harmonising and balancing massage may be particularly appropriate.

chamomile, lavender, neroli, tea tree, ylang ylang

Nerves – e.g. pre-exam nerves. We all suffer from nerves at some point, so help

chamomile, clary sage, lemon, mandarin, melissa, neroli

yourself to a calming essential oil bath to revive the mind and restore the spirits.

Shock – can follow any trauma, be it mental or physical. It may be linked to both hysteria and fainting, but is evidenced by shivering, a mental numbness or uncontrolled weeping.

lavender, neroli, peppermint, ylang ylang

Stress – for nervous tension, a regular aromatherapy is the ultimate antistress treatment.

basil, bergamot, chamomile, cypress, hyssop, jasmine, lavender, mandarin, marjoram, melissa, myrrh, neroli, rose, sandalwood, ylang ylang

Skin

Acne – caused by the overproduction of sebum from the sebaceous glands combined with bacterial infection. Commonest during adolescence, it can strike at any age and stems from a hormone imbalance or change. Massage of the area is particularly effective as it also helps drain the toxins away as well as combating the bacteria. For very bad acne a good hygiene routine is essential and a low-fat diet may help. Jojoba oil is the best carrier oil to use on acne-prone skin.

bergamot, chamomile, cedarwood, eucalyptus, juniper, lavender, neroli, patchouli, sandalwood, tea tree

Blisters – are caused by constant friction against the skin. Do not 'pop' the blister, but dab directly with lavender essential oil. If the blister is broken,

lavender

clean the affected area and dab with
neat lavender essential oil.

Bruises – discoloration and possibly
swelling which results from a bump or
graze. Initially the essential oils can be
applied in conjunction with an ice-pack
– add the oils to the water used to
dampen the cloth lying next to the skin.
Later, gentle local massage helps
disperse the blood causing the discoloration.

*geranium, hyssop,
lavender, marjoram*

Body odour – nothing is a substitute for
cleanliness and daily bathing, but these
essential oils can also be of use in the
bath or shower.

*clary sage, cypress,
juniper, lemon*

Burns – the body's response to too much
heat is pain, redness and possibly blis-
tering. The area should be cooled
immediately with ice or cold water. As
Gattefosse discovered, pure lavender oil
applied directly to the skin as quickly as
possible is the best treatment. Once the
skin is healing, gently rubbing a blend
of lavender oil and wheatgerm oil into
the area will further strengthen it and
help prevent scarring.

*chamomile,
geranium, lavender,
myrrh, patchouli,
tea tree*

Cellulite – the 'orange peel' effect to skin
which women get on their hips and
thighs is notoriously hard to shift.
However, aromatherapy is one of the
more successful methods. Massage of
the area stimulates the circulation and
encourages lymphatic drainage from
the fat cells.

*basil, cypress,
geranium, juniper,
lemon, rosemary,
tangerine*

Cold sores – caused by the herpes simplex virus that most of us carry round without any symptoms. However, the cold sores can erupt when there is another infection, or when the body is run down, overtired or under stress. Dab the cold sores with one of the oils in an alcohol base (you may be able to buy an appropriate alcohol from the chemist; alternatively, a small amount of vodka works well) or with neat lavender oil.

bergamot, eucalyptus, frankincense, lavender, tea tree

Corns – lumps of hard skin caused by continual pressure, normally found on the hands or feet. Rub the diluted essential oils into the affected area (an excellent excuse for a foot massage). Use corn pads to relieve the pressure and try changing your shoes regularly.

lavender, lemon, marjoram

Cuts (minor) – should always be cleaned. Essential oils are naturally antiseptic and so aid healing. Add a couple of drops to a small bowl of water and swab the cut. If travelling, lavender oil can be applied neat, but this does not remove any dirt particles which should be flushed away as soon as possible.

geranium, lavender, myrrh, pine

Dandruff – a scaly condition of the scalp exacerbated by the hair follicles becoming blocked with excess sebum. Add a couple of drops of essential oil to the rinsing water after using a mild shampoo.

bay, patchouli, rosemary, tea tree

Dry skin – skin which is lacking in moisture will benefit from a nourishing massage. Use a rich blend of avocado and wheatgerm carrier oils.

chamomile, frankincense, geranium, hyssop, jasmine, rose, sandalwood

Eczema – a common and distressing skin condition prevalent during childhood and puberty, and which is frequently linked to allergies or stress. Characterised by patches of itching, scaling skin that may produce a clear discharge if scratched. Often a good way to apply the essential oils is in a light, non-perfumed, aqueous moisturising cream as the carrier oils in some cases worsen the condition. For treating large areas of the skin and for small children, an easy way to treat the condition is by adding essential oils to the bath.

chamomile, geranium, lavender,

Infections – small unidentified infections can be washed in the same way as minor cuts.

eucalyptus, rosemary, sandalwood, tea tree

Inflamed/irritated/itchy skin – dermatitis is not a separate condition but literally means inflammation or irritation of the skin. The essential oils can help relieve the pain or discomfort – chamomile is especially effective.

chamomile, geranium, lavender, myrrh, patchouli, sandalwood, tea tree

Scar tissue – gently massage the area.

jasmine, lavender, patchouli

Sunburn – treat as for any other burn. If a large area is affected, lavender essential oil in an easily absorbed carrier oil topped up with extra wheatgerm oil would be better.

chamomile, lavender

Sweaty feet – an especially cooling and refreshing footbath is to be had with peppermint essential oil.

cypress, peppermint, tea tree

Ulcers – occur when people are overtired, under stress, or generally under the weather. Most commonly found in the mouth. These can be treated with a mouthwash of one drop of myrrh essential oil and one drop of peppermint essential oil diluted in half a tumbler of water, swill round the mouth and spit out.

eucalyptus, juniper, lavender, myrrh, peppermint

Warts – dab regularly with tea tree essential oil. Genital warts should be treated by a doctor.

lemon, tea tree

Note: The above remedy finder is intended as a guide only. If symptoms persist, consult your GP.

Glossary

Absolute – an oil obtained from the plant by solvent extraction. However, traces of the solvent may remain so they are not usually recommended for aromatherapy, but they do make an affordable alternative to some of the more expensive essential oils. Used widely in the perfume industry.

Antifungal – a substance which prevents and eliminates fungal infections, e.g. athlete's foot.

Antiseptic – a substance which fights infections and germs on the surface of the skin. All essential oils are antiseptic to a varying degree.

Base oils – see carrier oils

Carrier (or base) oils – the vegetable, nut and seed oils used in aromatherapy to carry the more concentrated essential oils onto the skin.

Diuretic – a substance that increases the flow of urine and reduces puffiness caused by fluid retention in the tissues.

Phytotherapy – a European term given to the use of plant remedies. In France, phytotherapy is a recognised part of medicine and is included in hospital training. Phytotherapy uses traditional remedies based on herbal extracts and essential oils.

Toxic – poisonous. Essential oils are non-toxic when diluted. The toxic essential oils are spice oils such as wintergreen and nutmeg and are generally unavailable.

Volatile – a substance which evaporates very quickly. The essential oils are volatile substances.

Useful Addresses

ACCREDITED PRACTITIONERS

Send an SAE to any of the following organisations for a list of locally accredited practitioners. They will also be able to provide the information needed if you are considering training courses.

The International Federation of Aromatherapists (IFA)
Dept of Continuing Education
The Royal Masonic Hospital
Ravenscourt Park
London N6 0TN

The Register of Qualified Aromatherapists
52 Barrack Lane
Aldwick, Bognor Regis
West Sussex PO21 4DD

Association of Tisserand Aromatherapists
PO Box 746, Hove
East Sussex BN3 3XA

London School of Aromatherapy, PO Box 780
London NW5 1DY

Shirley Price Aromatherapy
Essentia House
Upper Bond Street, Hinckley
Leicestershire LE10 1RS

SUPPLIERS

The following are suppliers of carrier and essential oils. Some also sell diffusers and other accessories. All of them run a mail order service or, alternatively, would be able to give you a list of local retail outlets.

Aromatherapy Associates
68 Maltings Place
Bagleys Lane, London SW6 2BY
(071) 731 8129 / 371 9878
(Excellent aromatherapy treatments also available.)

Bodytreats
15 Approach Road
Raynes Park
London SW20 8BA
(081) 543 7633

Fragrant Earth
PO Box 182
Taunton
Somerset TA1 3SD
(0823) 335734

Nelson & Russell
5 Endeavor Way
London SW19 9UH
Telephone orders:
(071) 495 2404

Fleur Aromatherapy
Pembroke Studios
Pembroke Road
Muswell Hill
London N10 2JE
(081) 444 7424

Shirley Price Aromatherapy
Essentia House
Upper Bond Street
Hinckley
Leicestershire LE10 1RS
(0455) 615466

PUBLICATIONS

The following publications are aimed largely at professional aromatherapists. However, they are very interesting and informative, especially as they cover new findings, legislation and developments.

Aromatherapy Quarterly
5 Ranelagh Avenue
London SW13 0BY

International Journal of Aromatherapy
(published by the Tisserand Institute of Aromatherapy)
65 Church Road
Hove
East Sussex BN3 2BD

The International Federation of Aromatherapists publishes its own newsletter for members (see previous page).

HOW TO ORDER YOUR BOXTREE BOOKS BY LIZ EARLE

LIZ EARLE'S QUICK GUIDES

Available Now

☐	1 85283 542 7	Aromatherapy	£3.99
☐	1 85283 544 3	Baby and Toddler Foods	£3.99
☐	1 85283 543 5	Food Facts	£3.99
☐	1 85283 546 X	Vegetarian Cookery	£3.99

Available from September 1994

☐	0 7522 1619 8	Evening Primrose Oil	£3.99
☐	0 7522 1614 7	Herbs for Health	£3.99
☐	1 85283 984 8	Successful Slimming	£3.99
☐	1 85283 989 9	Vitamins and Minerals	£3.99

ACE PLAN TITLES

☐	1 85283 518 4	Liz Earle's Ace Plan The New Guide to Super Vitamins A, C and E	£4.99
☐	1 85283 554 0	Liz Earle's Ace Plan Weight-Loss for Life	£4.99

All these books are available at your local bookshop or can be ordered direct from the publisher. Just tick the titles you want and fill in the form below.

Prices and availability subject to change without notice.

Boxtree Cash Sales, P O Box 11, Falmouth, Cornwall TR10 9EN

Please send cheque or postal order for the value of the book, and add the following for postage and packing:

UK including BFPO – £1.00 for one book, plus 50p for the second book, and 30p for each additional book ordered up to a £3.00 maximum.

OVERSEAS including Eire – £2.00 for the first book, plus £1.00 for the second book, and 50p for each additional book ordered.

OR please debit this amount from my Access/Visa Card (delete as appropriate).

Card Number ☐☐☐☐☐☐☐☐☐☐☐☐☐☐☐☐☐☐☐☐

AMOUNT £ ....

EXPIRY DATE ....

SIGNED ....

NAME ....

ADDRESS ....

....